icount™

10 Simple Steps to a Healthy Life

Caren –
to your health!

by

Susan Parks and
Patricia Bonavia

iUniverse, Inc.
New York   Bloomington

icount.

Susan Parks and Patricia Bonavia

iUniverse books may be ordered through booksellers or by contacting:

iUniverse
1663 Liberty Drive
Bloomington, IN 47403
www.iuniverse.com
1-800-Authors (1-800-288-4677)

ISBN: 978-0-595-52619-2 (pbk)
ISBN: 978-0-595-62671-7 (ebk)

Printed in the United States of America

Dedication

To Michael Levin and all of our wonderful family and friends.
Thank you for your heartfelt and healthy support.

Table of Contents

An Invitation

You count! You owe it to yourself and your family, friends, and employer to take the best possible care of you. You want to live long and be in good health to enjoy the fruits of your hard work and spend quality time with those you love.

If you're a CEO, a Human Resources executive, or a manager in any enterprise, public or private, people are counting on you. You owe it to your employees—and your shareholders—to find ways to introduce wellness into your workplace. The skyrocketing costs of healthcare and the lost time and efficiency due to poor health are most likely taking a huge toll on your company's competitiveness and bottom line.

Our country is in trouble. Health care costs are spiraling out of control and Americans are unhealthier than ever. There is a correlation. Health care expenses go down when people are healthier.

It's time to make a change, and it's up to you to do your part. How do you do that? By taking charge of your personal health and lifestyle, you can help alter the statistics.

The STAR™ Process

By reading this book, you will discover an easy method to Set, Track, Achieve, and Reward (STAR™) daily goals in the world of wellness. You will learn to do your daily wellness goals for three weeks to build a habit and ten weeks to become part of your lifestyle. From mastering simple, daily goals focused on you, you will create for yourself a healthier lifestyle that will have positive benefits in all aspects of your life.

This book is your guide and is organized into ten chapters each with a simple daily step that you can count on to achieve your healthy lifestyle goals. It will introduce you to your tools at WalkStyles.com:

- The Online Diagnostic Tool. Complete it after each chapter or at the end of the book.

- The Online Tracking Tools. Easily Set and Track your steps, nutrition, and other wellness goals.

- Your Online Dashboard. As you Achieve your goals, you will be able to chart your progress and Reward your success.

Before beginning any new exercise or nutrition program, including this one, you should consult with your physician.

Whether you're an employee or an employer, a homebuilder or a homemaker, a retiree or an intern, or anything in between, you'll find in these pages steps to take to achieve your goals in the world of wellness.

Say it out loud: I count!
Because you do!
So please accept this invitation to, as Aerosmith says, …
Walk this way!

Chapter 1:
I Count on My Commitment

Daily step # 1: Commit to my daily wellness goals each morning.
Process: Set, Track, Achieve, and Reward my wellness goals each day for 3
weeks and they will become my habits; Set, Track, Achieve and Reward them
for 10 weeks and they will become part of my lifestyle.
Healthy lifestyle goal: To live a long, happy and healthy life.

Why We Want You to Be Healthy

This isn't an exercise book. Or a nutrition book. Or a book about finding and enjoying the greatest relationship of your life. Or a book on how to be a better parent. Or a book on how to make more money than you ever dreamed possible.

There are plenty of great books out there on each of those topics. But most fail to answer one fundamental question: When you work for a living and when there isn't a free moment in your day from the time the alarm clock rings through fighting the commute, getting your work done, grabbing a bite for dinner and collapsing in front of the TV before you get some sleep, how do you find the time to do anything these books say?

We can set great intentions for ourselves, create inspiring goals, make New Year's resolutions ... but then reality sets in. We might want to make important changes in our lives—like adding a fitness routine or changing our diet or taking some positive steps forward in our lives—but then we bump up against the reality of time. All the diet, exercise, and self-help books in the world will fail us if we don't have the time to incorporate the changes they suggest into our lives.

If the time we have in the course of our day isn't growing, what is? Waistlines and health care expenses ... that's what's growing! Check out these alarming statistics:[1]

- 66 percent of Americans are overweight.
- 33 percent of Americans are obese (thirty pounds or more overweight).
- 70 percent of all illnesses are due to lifestyle-related causes such as obesity and physical inactivity.

And these figures are hurting individuals and businesses everywhere: obesity has been linked to higher medical bills, greater absenteeism, reduced productivity, and increased disability expenses in the workplace.

Here's another frightening fact: 40 percent of Americans participate in no leisure-time physical activity.[2] Instead, they zone out in front of the television or computer. What a way to live!

By contrast, when you're healthy, you can live a really great life… see your kids graduate and start their lives as adults…see your grandchildren grow up…maximize your effectiveness at work…and maximize your income, as well. It's not just about weight. It's about finding a way to take care of your health that fits in with the "no time/too much stress" lifestyle that we unfortunately face today.

The Solution

The solution is deceptively simple: we all need to become more active. Our goal is to help you find ways to do this and to keep doing this each day. As you'll soon see, the good news is that you're already on your way!

There are many reasons to exercise. A recent study found that people who walked thirty minutes a day had a 37 percent less chance of having a heart attack.[3]

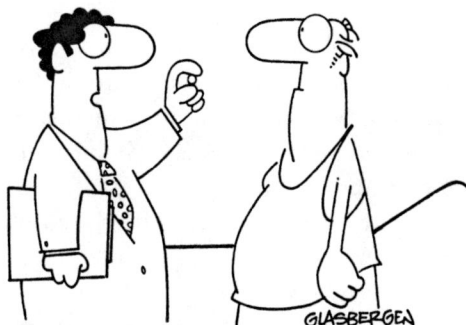

"To prevent a heart attack, take one aspirin every day.
Take it out for a jog, then take it to the gym,
then take it for a bike ride..."

Walking just 2,000 steps more each day can result in a ten-pound weight loss over the course of a year.[4] This doesn't even touch on the psychological benefits of physical activity. Exercise releases endorphins which diminish stress and make you feel more optimistic. Another study showed the link between belly fat and dementia and pointed out that when you reduce the belly fat, exercise being key in the process, the dementia risk decreases.[5] Exercising doesn't just work wonders physically, but mentally and emotionally too.

Of course, there are other things you need to do to stay healthy—exercise is just one part. But being active encourages your body to do other healthy things. Another study found that if you exercise regularly, eat fruits and vegetables, drink in moderation, and don't smoke, you can add up to fourteen years to your life.[6]

All of this is great news for you. But the question remains: How do you find the time to do the right things?

How We Can Help

That's where we come in. We aren't nutritionists or fitness gurus or MDs or psychologists, although we have all of these types of people on our team. We're businesspeople, and we have always worked for a living, just like you. We've never had time for elaborate fitness training programs or the preparation of complicated recipes after a full day of work. We have always

3

traveled a lot, which means that we spend plenty of time in airports and hotels, where nutrition choices aren't always the best and where temptations abound.

One day we looked at the way we were living our lives and realized that something had to give. It was up to us to find a way to stay healthy and fit, because juggling work and family demands was simply too much to manage if we didn't have enough energy. We knew that energy was a function of diet and exercise, and we became more conscious of our nutrition intake, but we struggled with how to get exercise time into our fourteen-hour (or more) workdays. How could we ever possibly incorporate a regular workout regime into such a hectic schedule?

When Sue had her first general manager position, she encountered more complicated situations than in her previous work roles and found herself needing to decompress. She started taking walks at the end of the day to think through the issues at hand, and after a while, she realized that the walking was keeping her fit as well as sane. A couple of years and several promotions later, Sue read about doing 10,000 steps a day. Originally defined in Japan well over forty years ago, walking 10,000 steps a day is a level of activity proven to keep one healthy, both physically and mentally.[7] She decided to adopt doing 10,000 steps a day, and in fourteen years, despite inclement weather, travel challenges, work, and personal commitments, she's missed only five days. By learning how to think of activity as a lifestyle, Sue has figured out how to fit those steps into every crazy day.

How did Sue know she was doing 10,000 steps a day? She considered a pedometer (step counter) the essential accessory for every outfit.

In Pat's case, she doesn't even remember when she started wearing a pedometer. It's been a part of her discipline and success for so many years, it seems like it's a part of her. It's no surprise that Pat, a highly successful banker, enjoys counting and tracking things ... like steps. In fact, one year she "paid" herself five dollars for every day she made her step goal, and at the end of the year she used the money to take her sister to Paris!

Because we lived in different states—Pat in Illinois and Sue in California—we challenged each other to online step-counting contests. This provided a friendly competition as well as a level of accountability we enjoyed and found helpful. What we both learned is that the power of Setting, Tracking, Achieving, and Rewarding our step goals was making us more effective in our executive roles. We had more energy and were tackling more complex issues with less stress. After a while, it became apparent to us that making our step goal was fundamental for our physical and mental health. This meant counting each step from the second we woke up to the moment our heads hit the pillow at night. We loved getting in a dedicated walk in the course of a day, but in many instances this wasn't possible. Yet we always managed to make our daily 10,000-step goal.

Sue remembers checking in at eleven o'clock one night in a Salt Lake City hotel and having the bellman watch her walk up and down the street. (This was before hotel exercise rooms were open twenty-four hours a day.) Pat would make sure her girls had done their homework and then would head to her treadmill with work documents to read while she finished her daily steps. We were always serious about making our goal, no matter how we got there. It may sound simple, but making our step goal each day was and still is the single easiest way for us to be healthy.

Why Steps?

Let's go back to the concept of 10,000 steps a day. The Japanese study conducted forty years ago demonstrated those 10,000 steps were the reason some people lived longer and healthier than others. There are other studies that reinforce the 10,000-step theory as well.

For example, a University of Tennessee study with pedometers revealed women who averaged more than 10,000 steps a day had 40 percent less body fat and waist and hip measurements that were four to six inches narrower than those who averaged fewer than 6,000 steps.[8]

In another study, researchers measured the steps of Amish adults with pedometers and found that the men took an average of 18,425 steps a day and the women took 14,196.[9] The average American takes about 3,500 steps a day. It's easy to see why only 4 percent of Amish adults are obese, versus 33 percent of the general population!

These studies demonstrate the power of achieving a daily step count (ideally 10,000) to reach and maintain a healthy weight. Excess weight, determined by Body Mass Index (BMI) or waist measurements, has been linked to cancer, heart disease, diabetes, back pain, dementia and more.

By now you've probably recognized that taking 10,000 steps a day is an excellent way to launch you on the path toward superior physical health, as well as a great way to improve your mental well-being. So how do you go about making a 10,000 daily step count a constant in your life?

The Process

The key to what we've learned through years of doing our steps is the importance of the goal-setting process. We've said it once, and we'll say it again: Setting a goal, Tracking your actual result, Achieving the goal, Rewarding yourself for the achievement, and moving forward is hugely empowering. What we've learned is that it takes three weeks to build a habit but if we do something every day for ten weeks, it becomes part of our lifestyle. This STAR™ process has enabled us to be healthy and successful executives who can still fit into our high school prom dresses!

Another study—this one performed at Stanford University—confirms our personal success stories. Scientists found that people who tracked their steps ended up walking more and gaining all the health benefits that come from this simple form of exercise.[10]

You don't have to walk 10,000 steps today in order to make this work for you. The good news is that, if you are like most Americans, since you are already walking 3,500 steps a day, you can start tracking something you've already mastered! Typically, those 3,500 steps are from the bed to the kitchen to the garage, from Starbucks® to the office, walking around at the office, to the car to drive home, and then from the garage back to the kitchen. Throw in the few steps that it takes to get from the kitchen to the TV or the computer, which is where most of us spend far too many evenings, and it works out, on average, to about 3,500 steps. You were already a third of the way to 10,000 steps before you even picked up this book!

> *Counting steps provides the easiest, healthiest, safest approach to getting fit, increasing our energy, and moving toward other health and fitness goals.*

Counting steps provides the easiest, healthiest, safest approach to getting fit, increasing our energy, and moving toward other health and fitness goals.

✮   ✮   ✮

Let's follow the journey of three people who are illustrative of individuals having different attitudes towards exercise and other daily positive goals. All of them want to be healthy, but two are consumed by the pressures and routines of everyday life. As we describe their lifestyles by step count, realize that some people substitute biking, swimming, running, or other forms of exercise and activities to reach 10,000 steps. It's all about getting more physical activity into your lifestyle—look at the conversion chart at the back of this book [Appendix A] or at WalkStyles.com for more information.

The three individuals we would like to introduce you to all work at the same company. Let's begin with Lynn, a single mom in her mid-thirties who has worked in the same office position for the last fifteen years. Lynn has slowly, but steadily, gained weight since her children were born. She is about thirty pounds overweight (as is 33 percent of the population,) and has had a recent health scare. Her physician strongly recommends that she change her eating habits and start exercising. In addition, when Lynn does have a minute to herself, she stresses about how to be a better role model for her children and about her future. She feels and looks older than she is.

If we were to track the number of steps Lynn takes each day, it would be around 3,500. Where exactly does she walk? Her steps are spent getting her three children up, dressed, fed, and dropped off at school; stopping for a cup of coffee on her way to work; going to and from the office parking lot; walking around the office; picking the kids up from school; and then making dinner, helping with homework, and dropping into bed exhausted. (Whew!) Lynn is just too tired to think of adding one more thing to her life.

Now, let's meet Joe. Joe is in his forties, and although he still sees himself as the fit high school football player he once was, Joe's waistline has grown from thirty-two inches to a snug forty inches. He averages about 5,000 steps a day or the equivalent thereof, so there is a little time set aside for exercise, as well as time for having fun now and then with the family and even some community service.

Joe's kids are not all that into exercise, but their thumbs are definitely Olympic-class, thanks to endless hours of computer games. Joe knows he should encourage them to go out and play more, but they love their computer games and are really good at them. Joe has started to notice that although his children have terrific hand/eye coordination, they are easily out of breath after a few trips up and down the stairs.

Joe is about fifteen pounds overweight; and, as you guessed, it's mostly around the waistline—enough excess weight to require a new wardrobe of clothes but, up until recently, not enough incentive to get serious about losing those extra pounds. Joe's family does have a history of heart disease (his dad died of a heart attack when he was fifty-two years old), and in the back of his mind Joe knows he should start taking better care of himself.

It is not bad being Lynn or Joe. But would we really want to look at our lives and say "not bad"? Why would we compromise in so many important areas? What if there was an easy, sensible way to "step up" to a healthier life?

Lynn and Joe could … if they took their steps up to the 10,000-a-day level. At 10,000 steps a day and with a few other healthy choices in their daily lives, they would drop those extra pounds. Plus, they would have much more energy for family, friends and work.

With more physical activity in her life, Lynn would start feeling better about herself and develop a stronger, more positive self image which would help her in her job and in her social life. Quite likely, her children would benefit as she would make healthier choices for them as well.

With a new passion for outdoor activities, Joe could get his kids out enjoying the fresh air and playing sports together. He would lessen his worry about his heart, knowing he was doing something proactive for his health.

With new goals setting tools, both Lynn and Joe could put a plan in place for their career growth. They could start delivering more projects in on time and begin assuming bigger responsibilities; thus, earning bigger paychecks. Lynn and Joe are just 6,500 and 5,000 daily steps away, respectively, from making significant changes in their lives!

Now let's meet Andrea. Andrea tracks—you guessed it—10,000 steps a day. How? Well, she's the CEO of the company that employs both Lynn and Joe. She gets in a lot of those 10,000 daily steps by walking around the offices of the company and the nearby factory, seeing how people are doing and finding out what's really going on. As CEO, Andrea makes much more money than Lynn's and Joe's salaries combined. When Andrea's family takes a vacation, they go to a first-class resort or Europe or on an adventure trip like an African safari. Wherever they go, they are active.

In addition to their exciting vacations, both Andrea and her husband are deeply involved in community service, serving on the board of several local charities that deal with issues close to their hearts. Their two kids are fit and are also good students. Andrea's weight, blood pressure, waist measurement, BMI (body mass index), and stress level are all optimal, thanks to healthy diet and exercise. No surprise there! You won't be surprised either to learn that Andrea is very goal oriented. She sets her goals and tracks how she is doing in almost all aspects of her life.

Who would you rather be—Lynn, Joe, or Andrea?

It may seem as though Andrea's life is unattainable, or even unimaginable, for most Americans. But it's not, because the doors of opportunity and advancement are not just open to only a chosen few. Andrea's parents never graduated from college, but they stressed education, family, health, and having goals. There weren't any handouts in life—everything Andrea got, Andrea earned.

This doesn't stop some people from looking at Andrea and saying, "Some people have all the luck."

✶   ✶   ✶

You've probably figured out that it's not about luck. It's about taking and tracking steps ... literally ... to making your dreams come true. Again, this book isn't primarily about diet and exercise. Instead, it's a book about lifestyle and making choices. Few of us, given the choice of being average, above average, or extraordinary, would pick average. But in fact, too many of us end up living average lives because of the choices we make. If we're going to have an above-average life, let alone an extraordinary one, only we can make that decision for ourselves.

And that's why this chapter begins, "I count on my commitment." That's because in your life, you count, you rock, you rule. Say it out loud. Go ahead, say: "I count! I rock! I rule!" Say it every day and mean it. We all want to make choices every day that lead to better results when it comes to our appearance, our fitness, our energy level, our financial life, our work life, and everything else. Again, the problem is that we often don't know where to begin. Not everyone likes going to the gym or eating healthy food or any of those things that we know we're supposed to do. And those of us who work for a living have to find a way to incorporate health changes into our incredibly busy working lives.

In your life, you count. You rock. You rule. It's all about you...and the choices you make.

We can't always count on our doctors to be our "primary health care providers." That's up to us. We can't count on the outside world to create a healthy meal plan for us. We have to count on ourselves ... to take the best possible care of ourselves. And if we're going to make a change, just one simple change that can have enormous repercussions in every aspect of our lives, we've got to find a way to do it that fits in with our daily lifestyle and our many obligations at work and at home.

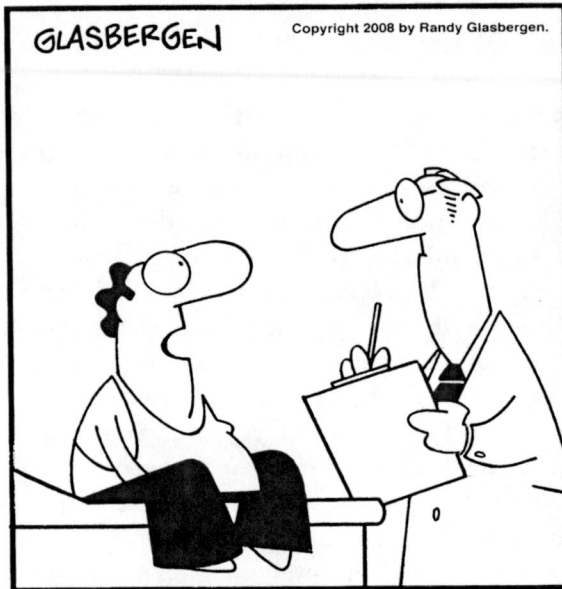

GLASBERGEN   Copyright 2008 by Randy Glasbergen.

"Eat less and exercise more? That's the
most ridiculous fad diet I've heard of yet!"

We're not promising you that if you get up to 10,000 steps a day you'll be the CEO of your company or all your health issues will go away. We can promise you that very few truly successful and vibrant people are able to attain that success without paying attention to their daily exercise and nutrition choices. There really is a correlation between how many steps we take and how great our lives can be. Again, it's about making a plan and having the discipline to keep it. Making a step count goal each day is a simple way to take control of your lifestyle.

Baby Steps

We understand that it's hard to make any change. We're not suggesting you to leap from wherever you are to 10,000 steps in a single day. We are suggesting that you Set a step goal, Track it, Achieve it, Reward yourself for making it, and then set a higher goal, track it, and so on. Start taking baby steps, and go up from there. If you add steps each week and work yourself up to those 10,000 steps a day, you'll lose weight and inches from your waistline. You'll have more energy. You'll feel better about yourself.

> *When you count on yourself to take care of your health, and when you count your steps, amazing things happen.*

You'll be healthier. Your relationships will improve. You'll find yourself more attractive ... and so will others. You'll be capable of doing more at work, which means that your compensation is likely to increase. When you count on yourself to take care of your health, amazing things happen. And it all starts with counting your steps.

Your commitment is key to the success of achieving your healthy lifestyle goals. Wake up each morning and make the commitment to that day's goals and you'll start seeing great things happen. If you use the STAR™ process with your daily goals for three weeks, you'll have formed a healthy habit. Keep doing them daily for ten weeks and you will have woven them into your lifestyle.

What's Next?

We're going to talk about the process of goal-setting from many perspectives in the coming chapters. In Chapter 2, we'll talk more about the importance of steps and how to fit them into your schedule and how they are the center dial of your personal dashboard. Once you start moving, good things happen to you physically and mentally. So, in Chapters 3 through 9, we discuss other aspects of your wellness, and you can determine additional goals you want to count and include on your dashboard. At the end of each chapter there are also diagnostic questions **(at the end of this chapter, you'll be asked if you are ready to be healthier)** so you can have a baseline of your wellness. This diagnostic tool is online at WalkStyles.com. At the end of the book, you will have an understanding of your current wellness, easy–to-use tracking tools, and your personal dashboard to keep you moving forward. You'll also be using a powerful process, STAR™, to achieve your daily goals and to help you reach bigger, important goals in your life.

The 6th-century Chinese philosopher and founder of Taoism, Lao Tzu, said, "the journey of a thousand miles begins with a single step." So let's step out together and start counting our way toward a happier, healthier, sexier, and wealthier you!

Online Diagnostic Tool Input:

Are you ready to start making healthier lifestyle choices?

★   ★   ★

Please go to WalkStyles.com to input your answers. You can enter and store your information after you read each chapter, or you can wait until you finish the book to submit all your answers.

Chapter 2:
I Count My Steps

Daily step # 2: Track my step total and aerobic time.
Process: Use STAR™ to reach a minimum of 10,000 steps each day and a minimum of 20 minutes at an aerobic pace 3 days a week.
Healthy lifestyle goal: Keep physically and mentally active for the rest of my life.

Expressions involving walking convey success. There's management by walking around, which our 10,000-steps-a-day friend Andrea practices. There are people who "walk the walk," or "walk the talk." That's something we admire. They've got direction in life. They've got a plan and a purpose. Many people refer to our spiritual lives as our "walk." The expressions surrounding walking imply that it's really a good thing.

Whether we were hunting or gathering, plowing or harvesting, our bodies were designed to be active. Now most of us have jobs or lifestyles that have us sitting at a desk, in a car, on a plane, and so on most of the day. The good news is that there are simple ways we can bring more activity into our daily lives just by being conscious of our step counts.

That's the beauty of walking—you're doing what your body was meant to do.

Our bodies truly were designed for walking. Exercise kinesiologists, people who study the way the body moves, will tell you that the best fat-burning exercises involve continuous use of any large muscle group. That's the beauty of walking. You're doing what your body was meant to do without putting undue stress on it! So, there's really no downside. It's enjoyable, and it can be social or introspective. It can be anything you want it to be. How you get your steps in is up to you. It could be walking, running, dancing, bowling, or something else. They all add up over the course of your day. Again, you can use the chart at the back of the book or our online chart to translate all non-step activity (i.e., biking, swimming, gardening) into steps. The real question is how to integrate the commitment to making your step goal—and ultimately tracking 10,000 steps a day—into your life.

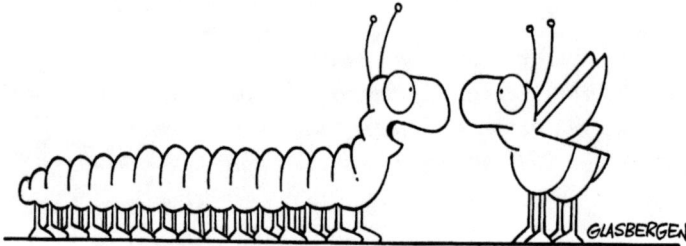

GLASBERGEN

"I tried all the fitness fads, but my doctor was right all along—walking is still the best exercise."

Take a Hike!

Okay. We are going to focus on walking, since it's usually the one thing we all do. It makes sense to build on that head start of 3,500 steps a day that you're probably already doing. You don't need a lot of new gear to go walking. All you need is a pedometer and a tracking system (we have the online tracking tools and dashboard at WalkStyles.com as well as a sample dashboard at the back of the book), a good pair of athletic shoes or comfortable work shoes, sunscreen, a hat or visor, and sunglasses. If you're going to walk indoors, you may want access to a treadmill—your own or one at a gym. However, you certainly don't need access to a treadmill as you can walk indoors in your office building or plant, a mall, an airport, your house, a hotel room, and many other places you frequent regularly. If you'd like information on Pat's and Sue's favorite healthy lifestyle products, you can see them on Sue's blog at WalkStyles.com. And, you can give us your feedback or tell us about your favorites too.

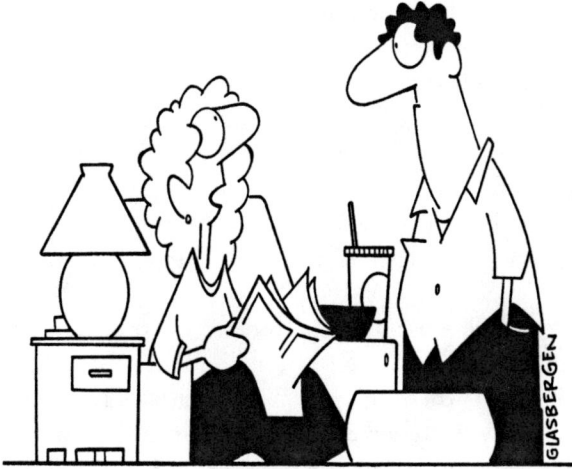

"I have a confession. I bought the treadmill
to cover a stain on the carpet."

The Device

Pat and Sue tested many pedometers through the years and were always on the lookout for a device that was small, good-looking, and accurate. Sue and her husband, Dennis, founded WalkStyles, Inc., and the company developed the kind of device we'd always wanted: the DashTrak®, an uploadable fitness monitor that combines features from a pedometer, a sports watch, and a heart-rate receiver. Realizing not everyone wants to upload, we introduced an affordable yet accurate pedometer, the Dash™. If you have another brand, great. We simply want to encourage you to wear a pedometer every day … from the first step in the morning to the last step at night. Wear it on your waistband or belt above your right knee. Think of it as your healthy lifestyle accessory.

One note about pedometers: wear a good one. We know people who wear one and say, it isn't counting right and put it in a drawer. You need to find the one that works for you. If you miss a step here or there, don't fret. You will get an occasional additional step too. Also, be sure to get one that tracks your steps, your distance and your calorie burn.

You must enter your stride length to get your *distance*. Again, don't worry that it is exact. Steps are what count, and a step is a step. However, you will want to know the approximate distance you cover. Just so you know, for an average stride length, there are 2,000 steps in a mile and thus, 10,000 steps is approximately five miles.

Finally, you will need to enter your weight to get your *calorie burn*. Taking the time to enter your weight is key because it is required to determine your calorie burn from your steps. As a rule of thumb, for a 180-pound person, the calorie burn is about 100 calories per mile. A chart on calorie burn can be found in the back of the book [Appendix B]. Pace can make a big difference.

To get started, wear your pedometer for three days and track your step count, distance, and calorie burn at the end of each day. Average the three days for each of these metrics. You'll start building your goals from these averages. **You will be asked for your baseline step-count, distance, and calorie burn at the end of the chapter and in the online diagnostic tool.** If you are currently tracking your steps at WalkStyles.com, you can select the starting point for your baseline online.

You may have questions on techniques such as how to swing your arms to burn more calories or how to work on your posture when walking. For answers to these and other walking technique questions, please visit WalkStyles.com.

Keeping Track

After finding your baseline step count, you will need to get serious about tracking. Again, you can do this all online using the tools at WalkStyles.com or create your own dashboard using the model at the back of the book. We even have a spiral-bound journal if you prefer. Just make a point of having a place to set this daily goal and a place to track your actual count results. Again, the process is to **Set your step count goal**, upload or check your pedometer each day, and then **Track your actual results.** When you **Achieve your goal**, be sure to **Reward yourself**, even if it's just to put a star next to the goals you have achieved. (Ideas for other simple rewards are listed in the back of the book [Appendix C].) After seven days of success, reset your goal (which will get higher and higher until you reach 10,000 steps each day) and move forward. Even when you reach 10,000 steps every day, you need to keep focused on the step-count dial of your dashboard. You wouldn't ever take your speedometer on your car's dashboard for granted, and you can't take your step-count dial for granted either. Achieving your daily step goal will help you stay healthy and fit for the rest of your life. That is definitely a reason to reward yourself!

From this point on, after you do your three-day baseline, you will always be wearing your pedometer and setting attainable daily goals.

There is a calculation you should know which gives you your Basal Metabolic Rate. To determine your BMR use the calculator at WalkStyles. com. These are the calories your body burns just from breathing and being. When you start wearing your pedometer, you are also tracking your calorie burn count from moving. The more you move and the faster you move will cause you to burn more calories. If you add your BMR and the calorie burn count from your pedometer together, you will know approximately how many calories you burn each day and that can help guide you to your eating choices that we will discuss in the next chapter.

Getting Your Daily Step-Count

Here are some tips to make your daily step-count goal achievable.

Think About It—*Never go to bed without thinking about what your day will be like tomorrow and how you can fit in your steps.* What opportunities will arise tomorrow to allow you to get in more steps? Maybe you'll have a little bit of time in the morning before you head into work. Or you'll be able to take a coffee break and get some steps in. Maybe you can take some or all of your lunch hour and walk. Or there might be some time after work.

> *Never go to bed without thinking about what your day will be like tomorrow and how you can fit in your steps.*

The beautiful thing about walking is that you don't always need to take time to get to the gym or change or hit the shower afterwards. Another great perk is that you can divide those 10,000 steps into multiple segments of walking throughout the day—you don't have to do it all at once. It's not about trying to fit your whole life around a new exercise program. Instead, it's about taking a look at your life and asking where you can spare a few minutes here and there to get your steps in.

Get Up Half An Hour Earlier—Our second suggestion: *If you set your alarm clock for just a half an hour earlier than when you normally arise, you'll be able to get in a whole lot of steps without disrupting the rest of your routine.* We know that doesn't sound like too much fun—getting up even earlier than normal. But it will only take you ten minutes to put on some workout clothes and get ready, and then you'll have twenty minutes to get steps in. You can do this outside or inside your home or hotel room.

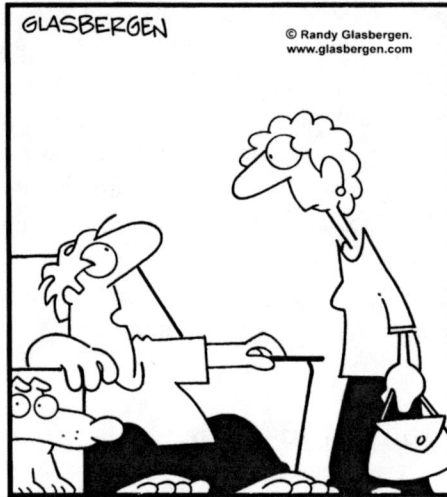

"I did a 30-minute workout today: 15 minutes looking for my sneakers, 10 minutes looking for my sweat pants and 5 minutes on the treadmill."

☆   ☆   ☆

In the first chapter, we talked about three individuals—Lynn, Joe, and Andrea—and their varied approaches to life. When it comes to alarm clocks, they all have different strategies. Lynn, our friend who takes the minimum 3,500 steps a day, is a connoisseur of the snooze button. Lynn sets an alarm on two different alarm clocks (one is never enough!) half an hour to forty-five minutes before the mandatory get-up time, allowing for multiple swats at the snooze. On most days, Lynn hits the snooze button six to ten times before finally dragging a tired, yawning body out from under the covers.

While not particularly buddy-buddy with the alarm clock by the bed, Joe at least respects it. Joe seldom participates in the snooze button dance; when the buzzer sounds, he is off to a running start. Okay, a walking start. But at least he is moving … even if somewhat reluctantly so.

Andrea, our 10,000-stepper, doesn't even use her alarm clock. Her body pretty much wakes itself up at the right time every day. It's remarkable, really: every morning Andrea rolls out of bed refreshed, alert, and ready for the challenges and pleasures of the new day.

Who do you most resemble?

✴   ✴   ✴

We're not saying you have to be a "morning person" in order to have a great life. We are saying that it makes a lot of sense to take advantage of the early morning hours … or even just a few more early morning minutes. Start your day with some extra steps, and you'll be on your way to 10,000 … and all the benefits that come from walking. In addition, your morning steps will help you make the commitment to all of your daily wellness goals.

Think Incrementally--We're not asking you or expecting you to leap in a single bound from wherever you are right now to the goal of 10,000 steps. We can safely assume that, if you're like most people, you're already walking 3,500 steps a day. So our third suggestion is this: increase your daily number of steps by 500 each week.

For example, if your baseline step count was 3,500 in your first week, then you would walk 4,000 steps each day in week two, 4,500 in week three, 5,000 … until you've gone all the way to 10,000 steps. Five hundred steps only takes an extra five or ten minutes a day, even for people who are not interested in walking very quickly! If you set your alarm clock to get you out of bed just half an hour earlier and walk for twenty minutes, you'll be able to get in at least 2,000 extra steps before you start the rest of your day.

> *Increase your daily number of steps by 500 each week.*

There's a lot to be said for getting in some movement or exercise early in the day. You actually reset your body's entire metabolism by moving and getting the blood flowing, so you increase the rate at which you lose weight … without having to put unneeded stress on yourself through other more time-consuming or difficult modes of exercise.

Many people are under the impression that to lose weight they have to run, not walk, and the faster they run, the more weight they'll lose. Walking raises your heart rate just enough to put you in the fat-burning zone. Working up to longer, continuous walks results in many of the same benefits as running with less strain on bones and tissue. Just one more reason to go the walking route!

Let's say you woke up half an hour earlier and devoted those extra twenty minutes to walking and got your initial 2,000 steps in. Add that to the "typical" 3,500 steps that the average person takes each day, and you'll be at 5,500 steps by just making one slight change in your lifestyle! Mix in a twenty-minute walk during your lunch hour and a five-minute walk during a fifteen-minute break and another twenty minutes after you get home from work … and you're at 10,000 steps right there. No sweat. No trouble. And lots and lots of benefits. Whether you jump 500 steps next week or leap all the way to 10,000 right off the bat, you're on your way to a healthier, happier, more attractive, and successful you. Additionally, you have begun a powerful way of Setting a daily goal, Tracking it, Achieving it, and Rewarding yourself!

Take Twenty-Minute Walking Sessions--Our fourth suggestion: whenever possible, aim for twenty-minute walking sessions. If that's not possible, go for ten, or go for five. Whatever you do is a step—actually, a lot of steps—in the right direction! But keep twenty minutes in mind as the magic minimum for as many of your walks as you can.

Also, make sure one of your twenty-minute walks is "heart-healthy"— walk at a slightly faster pace and get your heart rate up higher. This builds cardiac health and strength. How fast should you go? Fast enough that you can still have a conversation with a friend, but there should be some huffing and puffing. Fast enough that you'll know you've stepped up your pace a couple of notches. If you are using our fitness monitor, the DashTrak, it will calculate if you did 20 minutes at an aerobic pace and track it for you on your online dashboard. Work to increase your aerobic ability so you are doing a minimum of 20 minutes at least three days each week.

You'll notice that as you become fitter you will need to walk faster to get all your health benefits. We said that twenty minutes is the average time it takes the average person to walk a mile, or 2,000 steps. But we've also said that nobody wants to be average! If you speed up your pace, before long you'll find yourself walking fifteen-minute miles, which means that you'll be able to take 2,500 steps, not just 2,000, in the same twenty minutes. So now you have two ways to increase your efficiency—take more walk breaks, or walk faster.

> *Make sure one of your twenty-minute walks is "heart-healthy"—walk at a slight faster pace and get your heart rate up higher.*

If you have the time to walk longer, do so! If you did your 10,000 steps all at once at an average pace, it would take you one hour and forty minutes. If you added your normal day's steps of 3,500, you are now at 13,500! Now how cool is that?

Weather doesn't Matter--People often say to us, "It's all well and good for you to talk about getting out and walking. You live in Southern California, where you can walk outside year-round!" That's true for Sue, but she has lived this lifestyle while traveling around the country and also while living in Denver and Dallas. Pat lives and works in the Midwest, where winter is serious business, yet she and countless others still find ways to get their steps in.

We get our steps in on our treadmills, jogging in front of the TV, walking through airports or office buildings or wherever we can.

As we mentioned earlier, there's almost always a shopping mall or other indoor area that permits people to get in their steps, no matter what the weather's like outside. As long as there isn't a thunderstorm or an ice storm, you might consider putting on layers and enjoy the rain or snow for 20 minutes. At times, it can be refreshing or even romantic! So never let weather be an excuse or a deterrent to getting in your steps and taking the best possible care of yourself.

> *Weather doesn't matter. We get our steps in on our treadmills, jogging in front of the TV, walking through airports or office buildings or wherever we can.*

How to Spend Your Walking Time

So now the question arises—what exactly do you want to do while you are walking? How can you take what might seem like a ticket to boredom or drudgery and turn it into time that you actually look forward to every day?

We propose that, instead of thinking about your walking time as "the thing I've got to do in order to get healthy," you think about your walking time in these intriguing ways:

Think Time--In today's world of busy schedules and high stress, we're not really geared for introspection, even during quieter moments. Perhaps we're still checking our email or tidying up our desks or doing one of a thousand things that distract us from looking within. Think time is the antidote to the sense of hurry and the frantic pace that the working world sets for most of us today. This is your special time, a time when you get to be by yourself and with yourself and think through the important events and situations going on, not in the world around you … but in your world.

Work Time--If you have an appointment scheduled, why not do a one-on-one meeting while walking? You'll learn more about the person. Have brainstorming sessions. Nothing clears your mind or energizes you like walking. Or use your walking time to solve a problem. For Sue, walking initially started as a way to clear her head and come up with creative solutions to the management problems facing her at work. Many companies are encouraging employees with a disagreement to go for a walk and talk it out. Exhausted after a long meeting? Nothing helps get people back on track better than a brisk walk. Want to make a favorable impression on your fellow workers? Go see them in their cubicle versus sending an email! We'll talk more about this in Chapter 7—there's much to be said for being more active at work.

Doggie Time--Got a dog? Take a hike! There's nothing to keep you from taking your dog for a longer walk than you have before. Twenty minutes with man's (or woman's) best friend, instead of the five or ten that most dog walkers take, will give you a chance to bond with your pet as never before. And your dog will thank you for it.

If you love your dog, there is an even bigger incentive: much like people, 35 percent of the pet population in the United States is overweight or even obese. Just five extra pounds on a medium-size dog is equivalent to twenty-five pounds on an average woman.[11] These added pounds strain their hearts and cause other diseases, shortening life expectancy in much the same way that extra weight affects people.

Besides, your dog loves to walk … just say the word "walk" to him and see how he responds!

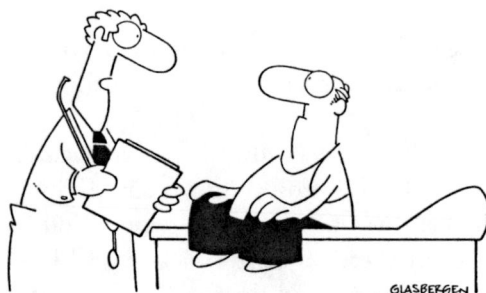

"Spend more time outside with your dog.
Teach him how to throw a stick for you to chase."

Family Time--Experience teaches us that our kids would leap at the chance (okay, leap might be a bit of an exaggeration) to spend twenty minutes of uninterrupted "quality time" with their moms and dads. Invite your children—one at a time or all at once—to join you on a twenty-minute walk each day. They'll get by without that extra computer time. You'll get a chance to connect more deeply with them, and you'll be modeling a commitment to fitness that all too many of our young people today lack. Childhood obesity is at an all-time high, and young people are coming down with forms of diabetes that typically were never seen except in people over forty. In fact, one out of three children born in 2000 will contract Type II diabetes, a form of diabetes that is directly lifestyle related.[12] So get out there with your kids and walk—it's a win-win situation all around.

Oh, and, like Andrea, don't forget that family vacations are meant for walking. What better way to see a town, a beach, or a forest than going for a walk?

Friend Time--When you get together with a group of friends every morning for a walk, you're really doing it right. That's because you'll be so anxious to discover the latest bit of juicy news, business update, or family drama that you won't want to miss a single day! Walking with friends makes the whole experience go by more quickly. We recommend it, especially in today's world where it's so hard to find or keep community. Find your fellow walkers … and hit the trail together.

TV Time: News Time and Silly Sitcom Time--Getting in your morning steps on a treadmill (or jogging in place) is a great way to watch the cable news channels and get informed. We call that "News Time." In the evening, when it's time to wind down from the day, it might be "Silly Sitcom Time"—time to just walk off the stresses and strains of the workday while immersing ourselves in yet another episode of *Seinfeld* or *Everybody Loves Raymond* or whatever you like. It's a lot better to watch TV on a treadmill or jogging in place than on the couch, for a lot of reasons. First, you'll be getting in your steps. Second, you won't be reaching for the high-calorie munchies. And third, after you've gotten in your twenty or thirty minutes of walking, you'll feel energized to go and do something else. Half an hour of sedentary TV watching ends up just making people want to watch TV for another half hour! And another half hour after that. And suddenly, the evening is over. So treat yourself to a half hour of sitcoms while you're on your treadmill or stationary bike or just jogging in place, because that will allow you to decompress and will energize you for whatever else you've got going on that evening.

> *Find your fellow walkers… and hit the trail together.*

Celebration Time--Who says you've got to celebrate birthdays, anniversaries, or other milestones standing still with a slice of cake in hand? Sue's friends have a great tradition: when a member of the walking group has a birthday, they walk the beach and celebrate with some breakfast champagne! You can celebrate happy occasions and achievements at work with a walk just as easily as you can sitting around a table. It's just more dynamic and fun this way. And there's nothing like starting the day with a walk and a bit of bubbly! Of course, this is for very special occasions only—if you were to start every day off with champagne, you'd be stepping a bit off-track.

Love Time--What a great way to talk through the events of the day with your spouse, relationship partner, or best friend. Personal time is so precious these days, especially given the demands of the modern workplace. Taking a twenty-minute walk with your lover is a great way to energize the two of you for your evening together ... and who knows where that energy might take you!

As you can see, walking doesn't have to be boring. In fact we hope you're starting to get excited about all the ways you can fit walking into your life. In the back of the book, you will find a number of our favorite ways to get in additional steps at home, work or on vacation [Appendix D]. If you haven't purchased a pedometer ... well, put this book down right now and either go online to WalkStyles.com or to a neighborhood store and get one. Your pedometer is your most important tool and trusted ally. Once you've got one, you'll be ready to rock and roll ... or rather, count and track!

We hope now you understand how easy it is to get in more steps. Walk more each week, walk earlier, walk faster, walk in twenty-minute (or longer) increments ... and before you know it, you'll find yourself at that magic number of 10,000 steps. The key is Setting a daily goal, Tracking, Achieving, Rewarding, and then moving forward.

So you now have your first three things to count and track on your daily dashboard. Each day, you will enter or upload your steps, your distance covered and your calorie burn from your steps. Those of you with a DashTrak® will also be tracking if you did your twenty minutes at an aerobic pace. You will define your own goals based on your baseline. Then, just start moving more each day. One small change, like taking your dog for a twenty-minute walk each day, can have a big, long-term impact on your health. Trust us, you will feel good making your step goal ... both physically and mentally.

So, what else should you count each day? Let's go to the chapter on nutrition. Because something you can count on is that the fuel you take in has a big impact on how you feel.

Online Diagnostic Tool Input:

My baseline daily step count is:
My baseline daily distance is:
My baseline daily calorie burn is:

Online Tracking Tools and Dashboard Input:

My commitment: Using the STAR™ process, I will always set goals and track my daily steps, distance, and calorie burn. (As a reminder, when DashTrak™ users input data online, the program will automatically track if you completed twenty minutes at an aerobic pace.)

Step ideas from this chapter to consider for the STAR™ process:

Taking a twenty minute walk each morning before work.
Walking with someone else three days a week.
Increasing my daily step count each week by 500 steps.
Walking my dog twenty minutes each day.
Others:

_____

_____

☆　　　☆　　　☆

Please go to WalkStyles.com to input the above.

Chapter 3:
I Count on My Nutrition

Daily Step #3: Track my food and beverage intake.
Process: Use STAR™ to eat a balanced diet and keep my BMI between 18.5-24.9; and my waistline under 35" if I am a woman, under 40" if I am a man
Healthy lifestyle goal: Have energy, feel good and maintain my ideal BMI and waist size for the rest of my life.

Your step count is the non-negotiable center dial of your personal dashboard; the only way you are going to make your wellness goals, both physical and mental, come true is by being active. Your distance is driven by your step count and stride length. And, your calorie burn is determined by your steps, your weight and your pace.

Consider this: You're focused to get to 10,000 steps a day. The last thing you want to do is undo all your hard work by eating the wrong things. We've found that people who wear their pedometers, make the effort to get up early, walk outdoors in good or not-so-good weather, take walk breaks at work, and attempt to enlist others to walk with them, don't want to undo all that hard work by eating something crammed with calories.

We've all heard the phrase "vicious cycle"—it's where one bad thing leads to the next. But how many of us have heard the term "virtuous cycle," where one *good* thing leads to the next? The diet and exercise industry is a multibillion-dollar business in our society, but it all comes down to one simple idea: lose weight by eating less and by exercising more. You're already getting the exercise in. And you're getting it in the most heart-healthy, fat-burning-efficient way—by walking. In addition, you've learned how to weave more activity into your daily lifestyle. So you've got the exercise part of the equation handled. The concept of the "virtuous cycle"—one good thing leading to the next—gives you the edge you need to stick to your commitment of eating healthier, because your body itself is beginning to reject the snacks that you wouldn't have thought twice about eating in the past. Making healthier food choices will not take extra time in your day. You only need to carve out 5-10 minutes to track your food and drink... it's well worth it.

☆   ☆   ☆

Where do our three friends fall on the calorie-count concept? Andrea can always tell you precisely how many calories are needed each day to maintain her weight. She also plans for healthy "breaks" and meals when possible and avoids "empty" calories and break room food. Joe knows that there are more calories in a muffin than in an apple, but he is still easily misled by his friends at lunch and many times picks up fried take-out on his way home from work. Lynn never seems to have the time in the morning to pack a healthy lunch and spends lots of extra time picking out her lunch and break food from vending machines.

But let's take a closer look to see how Andrea manages calorie intake and weight management. First, Andrea is aware not only of how many calories are required to maintain a consistent healthy weight but also how many calories are burned each day. This is because she always wears a pedometer, making sure that every day the goal of at least 10,000 steps is achieved. When she works off more calories than needed to maintain her current weight, she considers them "gift" calories and will enjoy a special treat or put them toward losing a couple of extra pounds in anticipation of the great vacation being planned by the family.

As Joe and Lynn started focusing more on their health goals, they began looking at ways they could make simple nutrition changes fit into their lifestyles.

Joe started with a rough idea of when too many calories were being consumed, but he hadn't determined the number of calories needed to maintain a healthy weight and how many additional calories would have to be burned in order to begin losing those extra fifteen pounds. His first action was to track everything he ate in the course of the day. That was eye opening! He had thought nothing of picking up several cookies while passing through the kitchen and eating them quickly while watching a game. In many cases, he wasn't even aware he was eating them. He was in shock when he saw in his food diary those cookies added up to 600 calories! He became disciplined in tracking his food and beverage intake into his daily online food diary.

Lynn had never been a calorie counter, but her recent health scare had her worried enough to look closely at what she might be able to differently. She made a daily goal of packing healthy lunches for herself and her children. They started planning the lunches together, so it has turned into a fun activity for all of them. Her daughter, liking this new energy from her mom, then asked Lynn if she would walk with her to school in the morning instead of dropping her off. Lynn called two of her daughter's friends' mothers, and they decided to take turns walking the children to school in the morning. This provided additional exercise which helped burn extra calories without adding additional stress to her life. Lynn asked and received agreement from her supervisor to adjust her work schedule to accomplish this. Lynn also started using her online food diary and was amazed at how many calories were in the coffee drink she took for granted each day. Thus, she decided to change her daily coffee order from a high-calorie mocha to a "skinny" mocha. She started noticing that the little changes she was making in her life were starting to have a positive impact on her and her family.

✶   ✶   ✶

So what should you ideally weigh? Obviously our bodies are different, and there's no absolute "one size fits all" approach to knowing our ideal weight. A simple rule of thumb is this: unless you're a Shaquille O'Neal-sized male, if your waist size is over forty inches, there's a good chance that you're carrying too many excess pounds. Same thing for a woman with a waist size over thirty-five inches. You definitely want to lose those inches for your health. You can learn more of your increased risk of disease by looking at our Web site or at the BMI (Body Mass Index) chart in the back of the book [Appendix E]. **You'll be asked in the diagnostic tool about your waist size.**

> *Unless you're a Shaquille O'Neal-sized male, if your waist size is over forty inches, there's a good chance that you're carrying too many excess pounds.*

Probably the best indication of where you are in terms of ideal weight for your height is to use BMI as your measurement of choice. To be in the normal range, your BMI should be between 18.5 and 24.9 [Appendix E]. You can easily determine your current BMI using our online calculator. **You will be asked for your current BMI in the diagnostic tool.**

Let's say that you've been getting your steps in each day, and if you aren't up to 10,000 steps a day, you're making great progress nonetheless. You now have the momentum, the edge, and the extra motivation to transform your diet so that you're eating better, eating healthier, and maybe even eating a little less than in the past. Just don't fall into the trap of thinking that dieting means starving yourself.

We don't advocate fad diets, crash diets, or doing anything potentially dangerous or unhealthy. Instead, we want to make it as easy—and enjoyable—as possible to lose excess weight and get healthy. Remember, this is all about your lifestyle!

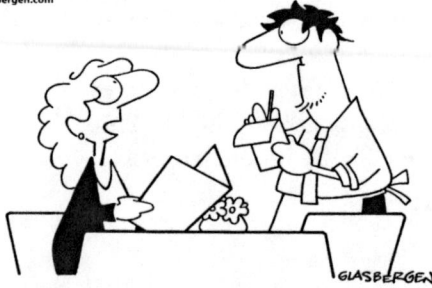

GLASBERGEN

"I'm going to order a broiled skinless chicken breast,
but I want you to bring me lasagna and
garlic bread by mistake."

We'd like to cut through the clutter for you and give you some simple guidelines about what, how, when, and where to eat. These suggestions are easy to implement in your busy schedule. These are proven approaches to healthy eating that invariably lead to weight loss, loss of excess body fat, and a healthier, more attractive you. The only downside is that you're going to have to deal with the increased attention you get … and you may have to spend a few bucks to buy yourself a new wardrobe when your old clothes don't fit! (A friend of ours likes to say that she has three sizes of clothes in her closet: small, medium, and chocolate … but that's another story.)

So here goes:

Know Your Calorie Intake Each Day

Don't cheat on your food log! You can use the simple food log and calorie guide at the back of the book [Appendix F], but we do have an interactive food log complete with calorie counts at WalkStyles.com. Much like you track your steps every day, if you want to lose weight, tracking your calorie count intake each day is very powerful. You will want to know the total calories you are actually consuming and if they are in balance by food types. You may want to consider adding calorie count to your dashboard if weight loss (or gain) is your goal.

You will notice that near your online interactive food log there is a place for recording your notes and thoughts. As eating and drinking in excess many times gets triggered by an event or by emotions, you may want to start journaling online so you can see what was happening the days your caloric intake goes higher than planned.

Eat Multiple Small Meals Throughout the Day

Who says you have to eat three meals a day? That notion came from a time when most people worked in factories; and, for the sake of order, they were trained to eat once in the morning, once when the whistle blew at noon, and once when they came home after the day's work. Today, we may work longer hours than nineteenth century factory workers, but we generally have a little more control over our schedules. Most athletes, personal trainers, and others involved in the world of fitness tend to eat five or six smaller meals a day. As a result, they rarely overeat, because they aren't subconsciously preparing themselves to go five or six hours until they see food again. That's why we say don't diet. "Dieting" implies eating less and has negative connotations of starving yourself. You may well end up eating less with this approach, but the point is that if you eat less food more frequently, you'll end up losing weight.

Be Careful of Outrageous Portion Sizes

This is probably the biggest issue with our diets these days. Muffins are now twice as big as when we were growing up. Same goes for bagels and most restaurant servings. Have some guidelines. A serving of protein should be the size of your palm or the size of a deck of cards. Use a measuring cup and figure out how much a half-cup of pasta or rice actually is. A piece of fruit is the size of your fist or a baseball. Whatever comparison works for you. Just be smart about portions. Don't hesitate to split meals in restaurants. Even if they charge you a little more, it is worth it.

Same goes for drink portions. You may even want to measure five ounces of water and pour it in your wine glass and mark the glass. Of course, this technique works with other liquids and quantities as well!

Take Pleasure in What You're Eating

It's all too easy to grab a bite over or near the sink when no one else is dining with us ... or no one else is watching. We recommend that you set a beautiful place setting for yourself. You'll be more respectful of your meal and of what goes into your body if you do. Who says you have to be with someone else in order to enjoy a meal?

We should actually enjoy what we eat! In today's incredibly busy world, most of us race through our meals and don't even notice what we're eating, either because we're distracted by other responsibilities or because we're eating stuff that doesn't taste very good. It only takes five minutes to put together a nice salad in the morning before you leave for work. The payoffs will be healthier food that tastes better.

Watch How Much You Drink

A lot of us have soda addictions—and we use the term *addiction* quite seriously. If you fall into this category, the suggestion we'd like to offer you is to replace those cans of soda with the equivalent amount of water. You can use the STAR™ process to start setting goals to drink less soda. One of our corporate clients has an employee who started a walking program and stopped drinking soda. In two months, she had lost ten pounds with just those two simple changes to her lifestyle!

A lot of times we think we're hungry, but we're really thirsty. Most of us go through our days—and therefore our lives—either partially or seriously dehydrated, and that's no way to live. There has been a great deal of discussion regarding how much water you should drink daily. Pat and Sue strive to drink eight eight-ounce glasses of water each day. Ask your physician for their recommendation for you. A couple of good tips: Drink water soon after you wake up, as your body will be dehydrated. Drink water before you eat, so you feel fuller … you'll eat less!

Don't drink unnecessary calories. Did you know that three large glasses of orange juice contain about 500 calories? That's one-quarter of the calories an average woman needs in an entire day! To get the benefits of Vitamin C from orange juice, enjoy an orange instead!

We (Pat *and* Sue) love our glass of wine each evening. As the saying goes, "All things in moderation." But we also use some of our "gift" calories from our steps to make up for this passion. Sue likes to think of it as a tradeoff: a glass of wine instead of a dinner roll. You can develop this technique as well.

Understand the Roles of Proteins, Carbs, and Fats

Most books on diet and nutrition spend an entire chapter on this issue alone. The main thing to know is that proteins provide the building blocks for long-term growth of your muscles, skeletal system, and other parts of your body. Carbohydrates provide immediate energy so that you can get through your day, and good fats also provide energy in a concentrated form, as well as transporting vitamins and protecting internal organs. Bad fats don't have a lot of redeeming qualities—in fact, they can cause some pretty serious health problems. Be sure that you are eating proteins, carbs, and fats in balance, and avoid fad diets. By using food log on our Web site, you can learn what percent of your diet is coming from each of the food groups and recommendations of changes you can make to eat a more balanced diet.

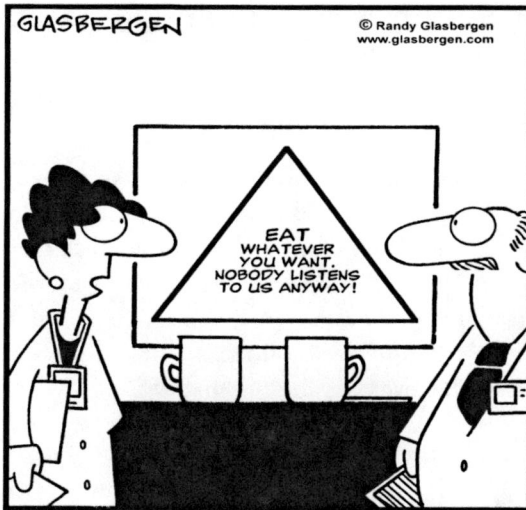

"They revised the Food Pyramid again."

Beware the Fattening Salad

Some salads have more calories than a full entrée because they're loaded with calorie-rich salad dressing and fatty items like bacon, cheese, and olives. Olives and cheese are great, but not when we eat them in excess or in combination with other fatty foods. Don't get into the salad trap. Instead, make sure that your salad really is salad—primarily or entirely vegetables—and use a low-fat or oil-and-vinegar salad dressing.

Good Fats are Good

Don't try to remove all the fat from your diet. Your body needs fat to function properly. Fat helps your joints work properly and gives you balance.

So taking care of yourself doesn't mean eliminating all the fat from your life. Most packaged goods now give you a label specifying the saturated fat and transfats. We provide this information in our online food log as well. Avoid these bad fats! You can get healthy fat from olives, nuts, avocados, cheese, and so on. Just be careful of portions.

Have fresh fruit for dessert most of the time but, on occasion, treat yourself to a delicious piece of cake or chocolate or a great homemade cookie. If you are having dessert, we recommend taking a bite or two of something really scrumptious instead of eating a lot of something average.

Five to Nine Servings of Fruit and Vegetables a Day are Essential

This may seem tough to do; but, portion sizes being what they are, you can do this easier than you think. In restaurants, order double vegetables. Have a big, healthy salad. Have a piece of fruit as a snack or as dessert. By the way, the darker the vegetable, the better it is for you--kind of like how dark chocolate is better for you!

So be sure to enjoy broccoli, kale, spinach, asparagus and other amazing vegetables whenever possible.

Never Skip Breakfast

Breakfast is truly the most important meal of the day. If you skip it, your body thinks that you're going into starvation mode, and it begins to slow down your metabolism, which means that you're not burning as many calories as you would if you had actually taken the time to eat breakfast. Skipping breakfast doesn't help you lose weight. It helps you keep the weight on.

Go For a Walk

When you have a craving for food, instead of eating it, go for a ten-minute walk. This is a wonderful technique, as you will likely forget about the craving after this brief exercise.

There's No Such Thing as "Blowing It"

If you eat a little more on any given day, either get in a few more steps or recommit the next morning. But never tell yourself, "I really blew it … so now I can use that as an excuse for eating anything I please."

Wise Choices

If you make wise choices, and savor what you eat, before long these new habits will become second nature. Use the STAR™ process to make small changes to your eating habits every day. At home you have absolute control over what you eat, and you can bring the right stuff to work—food that really satisfies you *without* pulling you away from your fitness goals. You can also eat healthy food on the road. Even if your only choice is a fast-food restaurant, you can generally find a healthy item on the menu. You may be surprised to learn that Sue eats McDonald's® food a couple of times a week. She just is careful to have no sauce or fattening dressings … and she rarely has the fries! Going to a fine restaurant? You can always order off the menu—they serve broiled fish and vegetables just about anywhere. It is sometimes easier just not to be tempted by reading the restaurant menu but to ask the waiter for the healthy option instead.

Let's talk briefly about supplements. There are certain things that you need in order to stay healthy that usually cannot come from food alone. Women, for example, need more calcium as they age, and it's tough to find enough calcium in even a healthy diet. So that's something you'll definitely want to supplement. And, just to be prudent, we think taking a multivitamin designed for your age and gender is a good idea. Of course, talk to your physician about your supplement needs. Just eat healthy, too!

Online we have sample menu plans for different levels of calorie intake as well as some delicious, easy recipes. These are all designed with your hectic schedule in mind.

Okay, now it's time to put it all together. At WalkStyles.com, you can calculate your BMI and know if you have a weight issue. If you are outside the ideal range, either high or low, you can start asking yourself what kind of tradeoffs you can make—in terms of walking, other forms of exercise, and nutrition intake—to get yourself where you want to be. You'll discover how many calories it will take to maintain your current weight and how many calories you need to subtract from (or add to) your daily intake in order to begin to lose (or gain) weight. Measure your waist. If you are not in the healthy range, you need to know you are at an increased risk of disease. You must count on yourself to do something positive for you. Start asking yourself where you can substitute a healthier food choice for a less healthy one. You can also determine what portion you can have of the foods you love, and still enjoy those foods without overeating.

> *You can also determine what portion you can have of the foods you love, and still enjoy those foods without overeating.*

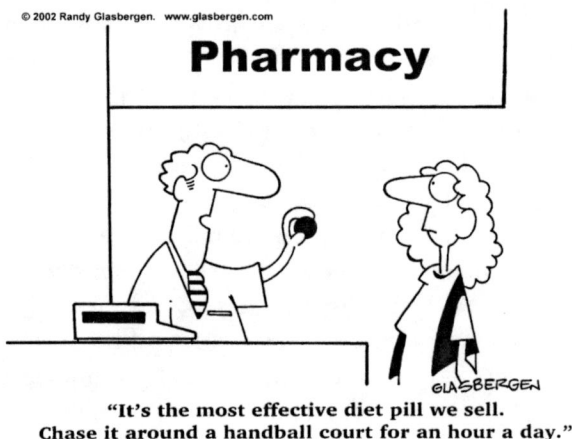

© 2002 Randy Glasbergen. www.glasbergen.com

Pharmacy

"It's the most effective diet pill we sell.
Chase it around a handball court for an hour a day."

It seems as though anything important requires effort and commitment, and that's certainly true when it comes to taking care of our bodies. We can make it as easy as possible, but we still have to do the work. Maybe that's the bad news. The good news is that your weight and your waistline *are* under your control … as long as you're willing to pay attention to how, what, where, and when you eat and drink each day. Use the STAR™ process to set achievable daily goals that allow you to develop a healthier eating style. Remember, changing just one thing you have been consuming, like one less cola a day, can have a big impact. Think about it in steps. Remember, you count! So start counting on your nutrition … today!

Online Diagnostic Tool Input:

My waist measurement is:
My actual BMI is:

Online Tracking Tools and Dashboard Input:

Nutrition ideas from this chapter to consider for the STAR™ process:

Tracking my food and drink input daily.
Setting a total calorie goal for each day.
Drinking eight eight-ounce glasses of water each day.
Eating nine servings of fruits and vegetables daily.
Taking my multivitamin each day.
Getting enough calcium each day.
Knowing the nutrition of the foods I eat each day.
Others:

_____

_____

☆　　　☆　　　☆

Please go to WalkStyles.com to input the above.

Chapter 4:
I Count on My Health

Daily Step # 4: Get enough sleep, sun, and use my common sense.
Process: Use STAR™ to get 8 hours of sleep and 15 minutes of sun each day;
listen to my physician and my body.
Healthy lifestyle goal: Live disease free and/or have my issues under my con-
trol for the rest of my life.

You've become good at tracking your steps and your food intake. What else should you count each day? You can set other goals—ones that concern your general health. Again, none of these goals will take too much time out of your day.

Walking improves your mental and physical health, as well as your overall mood. Exercise triggers the "chemistry set" in your body to fire off endorphins, which makes you feel good … which makes you want to get more exercise and eat better … which makes you feel better … and so it goes. Your brain functions better with regular exercise. You'll have less stress. You'll stay mentally younger … longer! Again, this is the "virtuous cycle" that walking offers, as opposed to the "vicious cycle" we looked at earlier.

One of the biggest concerns in domestic politics is the question of our health care crisis. Politicians routinely mention the forty or fifty million uninsured or underinsured Americans, and our government continues the struggle to find a health care plan that our society can afford. We're not going to get involved in that debate.

The easiest way to reduce your own health care costs is to get yourself a new primary-care physician. You don't have to look in the Yellow Pages or your medical plan directory. The best place to find your new primary-care physician is in the mirror. It's got to be you!

We have heard experts say that 50 percent of our health condition has to do with our lifestyle, and it's therefore under our direct and complete control. Twenty percent of our health relates to our genetics, and while we cannot do anything about our genes, we can certainly be aware of our family's health histories and be proactive with regard to any genetic illnesses in our lineage. The next 20 percent of our health is a function of the environment. We all need to be as "green" as possible with our daily choices. And, we can do a great deal about the health environment of our homes. The final 10 percent of our health care has to do with insurance, prescription drugs, hospital visits, and all the things that

America is desperate to figure out how to pay for. In this chapter, we're going to look at each of these four areas that determine our health—our lifestyles, our genetic backgrounds, our environment, and our approach to health care, and we'll see how healthier choices can result in increased health all around.

There are some key metrics for your health that you should know. For example, if you have high blood pressure, you should be working closely with your doctor. Your doctor has probably told you how beneficial exercise is for your blood pressure. One of Sue's friends, Muff, became part of the walking group because during a visit to her doctor, he told her that her blood pressure was too high. The moment she walked out of the doctor's office, she made a commitment to walking and lowered her blood pressure and lost thirty-five pounds over a six-month period. Muff used to describe herself as a third generation "couch potato." Not anymore! She looks and feels great!

Another friend, Irene, appeared to be in good health, but she found out some surprising news when she went in for her annual check-up. Irene's doctor discovered that Irene was borderline diabetic and directed her to reduce her sugar intake at once. With no known family history of diabetes, Irene was shocked. Having experienced the death of her co-worker, whose health issues were complicated by diabetes, Irene decided to make immediate changes in her eating and exercise habits. She reduced her carb intake, almost eliminated desserts, and added more fat and protein to her diet. She also began working out more and re-dedicated herself to getting 10,000 steps in everyday. After a year, she lost fifteen pounds, lowered her sugar levels, and now feels better than she thought was possible.

The point is, you need to know your own metrics and if any of them are out of the ideal range for your age, sex, and body type.

If you want to live healthy in our increasingly unhealthy society, you've got to count on yourself.

Lifestyle Choices

Let's start off with lifestyle. Most people who own cars take decent care of them. They change the oil every 3,000 to 5,000 miles, check the fluids, rotate the tires, and get their brakes adjusted. Why? Because cars are expensive, and most of us have learned from hard experience that it's cheaper, and less time consuming to do a little bit of maintenance than it is to bring a car in for a major overhaul … especially after the warranty has expired. Ouch!

If we take such great care of our cars, why don't we take equally good care of our bodies? Maybe because we got our bodies for free. If we had to make monthly payments on our bodies, or if we thought the way we treated ourselves might affect our resale value, we might act differently! The first suggestion we want to offer is that you get into the mindset of taking at least as good care of your body as you do of your automobile. You can always get a new car. But unless medical science accomplishes something that will surprise all of us, you get one body and one body only in this lifetime.

> *Get into the mindset of taking at least as good care of your body as you do of your automobile.*

   We consider getting regular medical and dental checkups a critically important lifestyle choice. Sticking one's head in the sand might be a great health plan for an ostrich, but it doesn't do much for human beings. The body is complex and often doesn't signal us that something's wrong until something is terribly wrong—as we saw with the case of Irene's pre-diabetes. Why take the chance? We compare regular checkups for the body to routine maintenance for an automobile. Okay, maybe there's a little less poking and prodding when you drop off your vehicle at the dealership. And they might even give you a loaner for the day! But unless we take care of our physical selves, we're buying trouble. Taking the time to get regular checkups will save you in the long run.

Copyright 2005 by Randy Glasbergen.
www.glasbergen.com

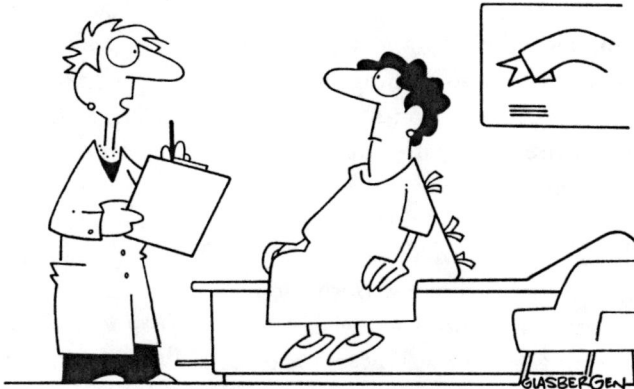

**"The only diet shake I recommend is the shake
your booty makes when you exercise."**

   How often should we go for scheduled preventive physical/wellness exams? UnitedHealthcare®, one of the nation's largest health care insurers, recommends regular preventive examinations for adults. The frequency of these examinations should be determined by you and your physician, based upon your unique needs, but here are some general guidelines for specific health concerns.

UnitedHealthcare® recommends periodic blood pressure exams for adults eighteen or older; periodic cholesterol screenings beginning at age thirty-five for men and at age forty-five for women; colon cancer screenings from age fifty; Pap smears for women annually until they have had three consecutive normal examinations, then every three years thereafter beginning when they become sexually active but no later than age twenty-one; and mammograms for women at normal risk for breast cancer every one to two years starting at age forty. Prostate cancer screenings for men are a matter that should be discussed with a health care provider starting at age fifty. While the US Preventive Services Task Force makes no recommendation for prostate cancer screening, the American Urological Association recommends such screenings. In between exams, it makes sense to perform appropriate self-examinations and screenings.

Not to beat the auto metaphor to death, but how many miles do you need to have on your odometer before it's time to go "up on the blocks"? **For the diagnostic tool, you'll be asked about your participation in routine physical exams.**

If there's a dramatic change on your body—a mole that grows or changes color, for example—you shouldn't need two corporate executives in the wellness space to tell you to call your doctor. It's a lot easier to allay any fears by getting the word from the doctor that everything's okay than carrying around the concern that something might be wrong. And you're not exactly doing a favor to your loved ones and friends by failing to have something checked out. **In the diagnostic tool, you'll be asked about how regularly you do self-exams.**

We've talked throughout the book, especially in the previous chapter, about watching your food intake. Obviously, we believe deeply in the concept of counting your steps each day. But it doesn't matter how many marathons we walk or run if we aren't eating properly. Physical activity and intelligent eating choices are the twin foundations of any healthy lifestyle.

> *Physical activity and intelligent eating choices are the twin foundations of any healthy lifestyle.*

Do you smoke? We don't need to go into details about this habit—there's plenty of information readily available, and today most people know the health risks involved. What we *will* do is offer a couple of suggestions. For starters, try using your new dashboard technique of Setting, Tracking, Achieving, and Rewarding. Why don't you track how many cigarettes you smoke each day? Then see if you can use an incremental goal to smoke one less each day.

Another suggestion: when you have the craving for a cigarette (much like a craving for an unhealthy snack), go for a ten-minute walk. Try it and see what happens. Again, it's likely you won't crave that cigarette as much when you get into this routine.

Need extra help? Go to the smoking cessation program offered by the American Lung Association®. We have the link on our site. We know it's a tough habit to break, but we want you to be healthy and happy! **You'll be asked in the diagnostic tool if you smoke.**

Do you have any other harmful habits? Excessive drinking? Taking prescription drugs outside of their recommended doses? Anything else? **You will be asked in the diagnostic tool if you have any other harmful or excessive habits in your lifestyle.**

Do you have any other medical issues? High blood pressure, diabetes, high cholesterol? Other? Again, this book isn't taking the place of your medical professionals but helping you with how you use a process (STAR™) to start making healthier lifestyle choices. **In the diagnostic, you will be asked if you know of any other medical issues. And, if so, are you treating them according to your physician's orders?**

Copyright 2003 by Randy Glasbergen.
www.glasbergen.com

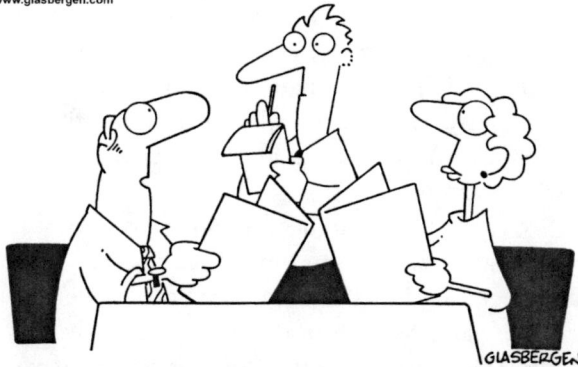

"I'll have some heart disease and high blood pressure with a side of clogged arteries and some tooth decay."

In addition to eating well, going in for frequent check-ups, cutting down on harmful habits, and treating other medical conditions appropriately, it's imperative that we get enough sleep. To see how much sleep you do need, please see the chart in the appendix [Appendix G].

Shakespeare said that sleep "knits up the raveled sleeve of care." Sleep relieves the mental pressure that builds up after the course of another day at the office. And it does a lot more than that. A good night of sleep allows our bodies to regenerate and to repair tissue damaged by environmental causes, hard exercise, and just the stress and strains of everyday life. We're putting an enormous burden on our bodies to keep themselves healthy when we are not giving them adequate rest. Sleep isn't a luxury—it's a necessity.

In fact, a study by the National Sleep Foundation in a survey of one thousand American workers found that:

36% have nodded off or fallen asleep while driving

29% have fallen asleep or become very sleepy at work

12% have been late to work because of sleepiness[13]

Another benefit of getting your steps in during the day is that you will be ready for bed and fall asleep quicker. Just don't vigorously exercise right before bedtime. **In the diagnostic tool, you will be asked if you get enough sleep.**

In the last chapter, we mentioned the importance of different vitamins, and in this portion of our discussion on health, we want to emphasize the importance of vitamin D. In our discussions with Dr. Eileen Hoffman, clinical associate professor of medicine at New York University School of Medicine, we learned the best way to get enough vitamin D each day is to go outside for fifteen minutes, revealing as much skin as reasonable. (Yes, we recommend you do wear something!) For the fifteen minutes, don't wear sunscreen. Even when it is cloudy, you are still getting some sun. Your skin is an organ, and it will absorb the UVB rays during sun exposure and produce vitamin D, which allows many of your other organs to function properly. Of course, we recommend you spend this fifteen minutes … walking. And, if you can't go outside for any reason, be sure your diet or supplements include Vitamin D.

Earlier we highlighted the need to spend twenty minutes walking at an aerobic pace, and we want to emphasize this in the health section. This twenty-minute walk will strengthen your heart as well as improve your overall circulation. Again, be sure to do all exercise only with approval of your physician. **You'll be asked on the diagnostic tool if you get regular aerobic exercise.**

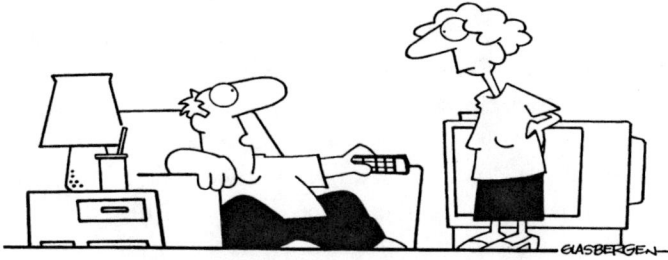

"My doctor told me to start my exercise program
very gradually. Today I drove past a store
that sells sweat pants."

Our lifestyles are a function of the choices we make. Fifty percent of our health is a function of our lifestyle. Taking control of your lifestyle and your health is a conscious decision, and it requires you to take action to make it happen. The healthier our choices, the healthier we live. It's that simple.

Genetics

Next, let's turn to the 20 percent of our health that we cannot control—genetics. We can't choose our families or their medical histories, but we can certainly be aware of what we may face. Know your history, be alert, and be proactive. A friend of Sue named Tom lost his mother and a sister to a brain aneurysm. For a long time, his daughter tried to convince him to go for a test, but he continued to refuse. His argument was that he was asymptomatic, nothing felt wrong, and if you had a brain aneurysm, there wasn't much you could do about it. Fortunately, his daughter prevailed, and she got him to take the test. It turned out that he had a bulging artery in the base of his brain on the verge of exploding. He had surgery to repair the artery, and he was fine. Did his daughter save his life? She set things in motion. Ultimately, he saved his own life by going in for the test. **In the diagnostic tool, you will be asked if you know your family health history.**

☆　　☆　　☆

Let's take a minute to check on how Andrea, Joe, and Lynn take care of their personal health. Due to Lynn's health concern, she arranged to meet with the Human Resources Department to better understand the company's health coverage. She was unaware that the company paid employees for the time they took to visit the doctor for annual physicals and dental checkups. She decided to make appointments for the entire family and, by the way, began taking one of her breaks as a "walking break," which increased her steps by an additional 500 per day, bringing her up to 5,500 steps on most days! Joe and his wife decided to cut back on the number of fried foods they consumed a week and began taking walks with the kids and dog after dinner three times a week. Joe also spoke with his mother to determine if his father's heart condition was due to lifestyle or was an issue in his father's family. He realized his father led an inactive life, and Joe is determined to be around to get to know his grandkids. He is up to 7,000 steps a day!

Meanwhile, Andrea has been encouraging the employees to attend the company's upcoming health fair and to invite family members to join them. She has given each of her employees two hours off during the day to attend the fair and has some fun incentive rewards for the employees who go to each booth.

✫　　✫　　✫

Our Environment

Now let's turn to the question of the environment. Collectively, our society—and on a larger scale, the world—is moving toward a better understanding of global warming, depletion of natural resources, and other critical issues that will hopefully be addressed quickly and effectively.

One of the most important environments affecting us is that of our own home. Since 20 percent of our health is a function of our environment, it's up to each of us to make sure that we live in and maintain a healthy environment for ourselves. For one thing, this means we want to make absolutely sure that there is no lead paint in our home (including in our children's toys). We want to have our homes tested for asbestos and radon to make sure that we, our children, and even our pets are not exposed to harmful chemicals and substances. We need to know what substances or potentially dangerous chemicals our family is coming in contact with, and we need to live in a more environmentally alert manner. We also suggest taking time to reduce the clutter in your home. You'll get steps in cleaning and, mentally, you'll feel great by recycling or donating the things you don't use or need any more. You may have to set aside some extra time on the day you clean but knowing where everything is will save you countless hours of searching.

Is there positive energy in your home? In Chapter 6, we will talk about surrounding yourself with people who believe in healthy lifestyles. In Chapter 8, we emphasize the need of setting some time aside just for you.

In the diagnostic tool, you will be asked if you are confident you have a healthy home environment.

Health Care

So far in this chapter, we've talked about 90 percent of the factors that influence our health—the 50 percent that is lifestyle and the 20 percent each represented by genes and the environment. Now it's time to face the final 10 percent; the question of health care coverage. This includes your health insurance, your level of benefits, and any medications that you or your loved ones may need.

If you're reading this book, you probably have health care insurance—you're either covered by your employer or you are self-employed and purchase your own. So the real question isn't whether you have it or not, it's this: What are you doing with your plan? Do you understand all the terms? Plans change every year, as providers and employers renegotiate their deals. If you understand your plan, are you getting all the benefits to which you are entitled? If the plan offers regular physical and dental checkups, are you getting them? Have you used your plan to establish a relationship with a doctor you like and trust, one to whom you can address candid questions? Some more questions for you to ponder: Do you have a health savings account (HSA)? If so, do you know what good it can do for you? How can you benefit from your HSA, and how does it fit into your overall personal financial plan? If you don't know the answers, don't be embarrassed. You're not alone. But it's time to scope them out. **In the diagnostic tool, you will be asked if you know the details of your health care plan.**

Childhood Obesity

It's essential for us to take the best possible care of ourselves, not just for our own sakes, but because the next generation is watching. What and how much we eat and how much we exercise influence not only our own health but also the health of our children. And the reality is that we Americans aren't doing a very good job of being good role models. The greatest new health crisis in American society is childhood obesity, now approaching an alarming rate of 18 percent of all children.[14] And for kids born in the year 2000, the news is especially bleak—they represent the first generation expected to live a shorter lifespan than their parents and grandparents. Remember, of children born in the twenty-first century, a shocking one in three will develop Type II diabetes.[15] We've got to take care not just

> *We have to count on ourselves for our health, because there is no one else in the world—not our doctors, not our parents, no one—who has nearly as much power to influence our health and wellness as we do.*

of ourselves but of our children if we are to be loving parents and responsible members of society. Kids need one hour of activity per day. Let them run and play! And "virtual" running—say, a video game character running onscreen while your child sprawls out on a bean bag on the floor—doesn't count.

The bottom line: we have to count on ourselves for our health, because there is no one else in the world—not our doctors, not our parents, no one—who has nearly as much power to influence our health and wellness as we do. And now more than ever, our kids are counting on us to make the right health choices, too.

The good news is that everything gets easier when you have a process—even taking responsibility for our own health. Initially, when you started moving toward 10,000 steps a day, it might have seemed like an impossible task. But little by little, you are getting there! Same thing with the diet suggestions we offered in the previous chapter. They may seem like a lot—especially all at once—but by layering in a few and then a few more, you will be able to build on the momentum that walking created and increase your vitality while decreasing your weight. Before long, in fact, it will become almost effortless. We're certain that when you take command of your health the same way you've taken command of your exercise and diet, the results are going to be exhilarating. Just start using the STAR™ process. We know you'll thank yourself for it … and so will your family!

Just one small daily change, like getting fifteen minutes of sun a day, can make a huge impact on your health. So … if you're willing to take control of your lifestyle and count on your health as never before … Setting goals, Tracking your progress, Achieving great results, and Rewarding your success, then don't just give yourself a STAR … recognize that you ARE a STAR!

Online Diagnostic Tool Input:

Are you current on your regular exams (medical and dental)?
Are you current on your self exams?
Do you smoke?
Do you overuse alcohol or other substances?
Do you have other medical issues, and, if so, are you treating them according to your doctor's instructions?
Do you get enough sleep each night?
Do you get twenty minutes of aerobic activity regularly?
Do you know your family medical history?
Is your home free of toxins?
Do you know your health care plan?

Online Tracking Tools and Dashboard Input:

Health ideas from this chapter to consider for the STAR™ process:

Getting fifteen minutes of sunlight (or vitamin D equivalent) each day.
Walking at an aerobic pace for 20 minutes five times per week.
Sleeping eight hours each night.
Others:

_____

_____

☆ ☆ ☆

Please go to WalkStyles.com to input the above.

Chapter 5:
I Count on My Strength

Daily Step # 5: Do my strength exercises.
Process: Use STAR™ to do a minimum of 4 strength exercises working up to a minimum of 20 minutes each day at least 3 days a week.
Healthy lifestyle goal: Have strong bones, muscles and good posture for the rest of my life.

How strong are you?

It's all too easy to neglect core strength and focus only on cardiovascular strength. Walking gives you a great way to build the strength of your heart, your lungs, and your walking muscles. And it's actually a weight-bearing exercise, so it does add to your core fitness. But walking alone is not enough to develop the strong muscles and bones you need for maximum endurance and energy right now and for later on in life, so that you can avoid age-related issues like brittle bones and loss of height—both signs of osteoporosis.

It's hard to convince people in their twenties and thirties that one day they will be older and the decisions they make now with regard to developing and maintaining physical strength will make a life-and-death difference. But it's true. We know a woman in her early fifties, whom we'll call Julie, who, when younger, never developed much of an interest in eating right or working out. Like most people, she thought she would stay young forever. One morning when she was fifty-two, she went outside to start her car. She reached for the gearshift, started to move it, and broke a bone in her hand.

Another woman we know, Sarah, also had never developed an appetite for strength-building exercises or eating healthy. She was a runner, and she figured that the cardiovascular benefits she attained from running would be sufficient for every aspect of her physical well-being, now and in the future. Wrong. One time while running, she tripped ... and broke her pelvis. Sarah wasn't in her seventies or eighties, the age when this kind of thing becomes more common. Sarah was also in her early fifties.

The moral of the story is simple: we can pay a big price for neglecting the strength of our bones and our muscles, incredibly important aspects of self-care. As a contrast to the experiences of Julie and Sarah, we'd like to tell you about Sheila, who owns the legendary Oaks at Ojai spa. Recently, we saw her speak on a panel about physical fitness. During the twelve minutes she spoke, she actually performed sixty-seven push-ups, to the amazement of the crowd. Sheila is not in her twenties. In fact she's not in her thirties, forties, or even her fifties or sixties. Sheila is in her mid-to- late seventies! We're certain that she could easily do as many push-ups as she is years of age. Not too many people of any age, aside from an officer in the Marines, can make a statement like that.

> *While it may not be true that only the strong survive, the strong are far more likely to thrive.*

Why do we need to be physically strong? Life takes energy. Everything you want to do, and do well, takes a considerable investment of energy, from your work life to your love life, from the raising of children to the raising of your net worth. As we saw in the first chapter, while it may not be true that only the strong survive, the strong are far more likely to thrive. A recent study put participants through nine months of regular strength-training exercises. At the end of that time, they demonstrated an average **22 percent improvement in their physical fitness … and a 70 percent increase in their ability to make complex decisions.**[16]

Whether it's avoiding medical problems down the line, maximizing our energy and our enjoyment of life today, or a combination of the two, there's a great case to be made for strength training. In many cases, this makes people think they need to join a health club but they lack motivation and time.

We can definitely relate to gym woes and phobias. Not everybody's a gym rat! A lot of us don't like to come in contact with, or even smell, other people's sweat. Others don't like the gym because they feel intimidated by some of the beautiful bodies, female and male, that they see there. We think men are just as uncomfortable as women in this regard. We women have a hard time seeing younger women walking around the gym in tight little spandex outfits. Men seem to have no problem with *that,* but they often find it uncomfortable to be in the presence of younger, fitter, stronger guys. They'll never say so, but we know it's true!

On top of that, exercise just seems so complex and time-consuming. Open any book on health and fitness and you're likely to find dozens of diagrams of exercises, all of which look complicated and most of which look painful. Not much fun in that. Also, and think about this, we tend to think of exercise as something we have to go to, so it does take extra time … and who has that? It is ironic that we have more gyms and health clubs than ever, and the country is heavier and out of shape like never before. Hmmm. How do you work through all of the exercise options and come up with a program that gets you where you want to go?

☆　　☆　　☆

Andrea would answer the question for us, but we'd have to find her on her exercise mat first. She has strength exercise as a goal she tracks on her dashboard each day.

Joe has always been interested in exercise … he still talks about his high school football days. On the positive front, he has started parking as far away as possible from the office building and has begun walking to the deli at lunch. He is up to 8,000 steps a day! Give me a J … give me an O … give me an E …!

Lynn has never been too much into exercising, but she has been motivated to improve her life, and give up one of her breaks to walk with another co-worker, who also wants to drop a few pounds and feel better. She also started a fun game at home with her kids. They have a contest of who can do the most jumping jacks during a commercial. Lynn makes sure one of her children always wins!

☆   ☆   ☆

As executives running a business in the area of corporate wellness, we've had to spend a great deal of time addressing this issue—not just for our clients but also for ourselves. We've come up with four exercises—not fourteen, not forty, but four simple exercises that you can do just about anywhere, without a gym, without spandex, without anyone looking, without equipment, and without leaving the comfort of your home or hotel room. If you work these four activities into your life on a regular basis, you'll be amazed at how quickly and effectively your body transforms itself into a powerhouse of physical strength. Okay, you might not be ready to join the World Wrestling Federation®, but that's probably not on your list of lifetime goals anyway. If you're like most people, you want to be strong enough to do what we talked about earlier—have a healthy lifestyle now and avoid illness and accidents later on. So let's talk about how to do just that. **For the diagnostic tool, you'll be asked to report how many repetitions of these exercises you can do right now.** This is your baseline. Remember, don't cheat and don't hurt yourself! For more details on these four and other exercises, stretching techniques, breathing recommendations and more, please go to WalkStyles.com.

> *If you work these four activities into your life on a regular basis, you'll be amazed at how quickly and effectively your body transforms itself into a powerhouse of physical strength.*

Exercise Number One: The Squat

It's easy, it's efficient, and you can probably do more than you realize right now. Squats strengthen your bone structure and aid your core fitness. There are few things more important in life than having a strong core, because this is the part of your body that allows you to do just about everything from swinging a tennis racket or a golf club to picking up your kids to hoisting a heavy package or a piece of furniture on your shoulder (if you're so inclined!). Core fitness is a huge buzz term, so you will be absolutely *au courant* with all of the fitness trainers and workout aficionados. And soon you'll be right up there with the rest of them.

The best way to do a squat is simply to stand against a wall with your legs extended out, adjusting your knees so that when you bend and straighten, you feel no pain in your knees. Breathing deeply, bend your knees to slide your back down the wall. If you can, you should squat until you're practically in a sitting position, rise up to standing position again, and repeat the process (you can do more, as you grow stronger). If there isn't a wall that's readily accessible, that's fine: do it without one. Squats are the perfect exercise because they build both strength and core fitness. They're great for the legs, behind, and stomach, too. No special exercise equipment necessary.

When do you do squats? Sue does them when she brushes her teeth! She says it may sound dorky, but this way the squats don't take any more time out of her day. She's able to do fifteen squats while brushing each side of her teeth top and bottom, so she does sixty squats morning and night—120 squats a day. As a result, Sue has strong bones ... and fresh breath, besides!

Exercise Number Two: Leg Lifts

How about doing leg lifts instead of snack curls and soft drink elbow-bending while you watch TV? Here's how: Lie down on the carpet (or even an exercise mat) and keep your back flat against the floor. Hold your stomach in and lift your legs so you are forming an L. Lower your legs, keeping them straight, but don't quite touch the floor, and lift again. It may help for you to put your hands under your behind. Leg lifts allow you to work your abs, your stomach muscles, and your core fitness.

Exercise Number Three: The Push-up

As with all these exercises, don't worry if you can only do one right now. Tomorrow, aim to add one more. And then another one the next day, and so on. Sue says she was once able to do twelve push-ups at a party, and people were very impressed! Now she can do thirty-five. You probably want her at your next party, as she is such a fun guest! The more you do, the easier they get, the stronger you become, and the better you feel about yourself. So there's a lot to say for the push-up. Granted, it's not the latest cutting-edge Pilates technique. But it's a powerful way to increase your fitness and core strength. You probably know how to do them: Lie face down; put your feet together and your toes on the ground, heels up. Place your hands shoulder width apart on the ground. Keep your core straight and push up! You can modify them (be on your knees) if necessary.

Exercise Number Four: The Crunch

Lie flat on the carpet or an exercise mat. Place your feet flat on the floor so your knees are pointing up. Place your hands behind your head or neck, but don't push with your hands. Allow your core to tighten and at the same time, lift your head and shoulders as well as your legs. See how many you can do right now, and commit to doing more each day. This works your upper abdominal muscles and gives nice shape and definition to your stomach.

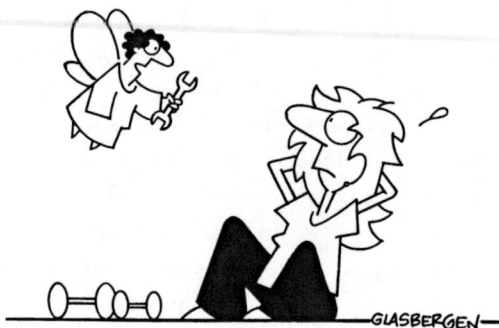

©Randy Glasbergen.
www.glasbergen.com

GLASBERGEN—

**"I'm the Workout Fairy.
I'm here to tighten your abs!"**

So there you have it—four exercises, as simple as can be. Squats, leg lifts, push-ups, and crunches. And since the magic number in this book is twenty, work your way up to twenty minutes a day with five minutes devoted to each exercise. Strive to do three sets of twenty repetitions of each of these exercises. Again, pace yourself. It is about continual improvement. And if you have the time, there are more exercises on our Web site working on specific parts of your body, as well as tips on stretching and other techniques. We like these four basic exercises because we know you can work them into your daily lifestyle.

> *It is about continual improvement.*

You'll be in better shape before you know it. Don't try to push yourself too much and hurt yourself. Start with just a few, perhaps even twenty seconds' worth instead of twenty minutes' worth, and watch how they add up. Use your STAR™ process and see your strength build!

Let's say that you'd like to go beyond these four exercises and actually get involved at a gym. We say great! Gyms and health clubs have a social aspect that can positively affect your commitment to exercise. You can have fun meeting people in addition to getting a workout. Group exercise classes tend to push people to work harder than they would on their own, and you can find everything from yoga and Pilates to more traditional gym fare like aerobics classes and spinning. The accountability of meeting a friend or a trainer at a gym is also powerful motivation to increase your level of fitness.

If you want to know how to get started in the gym or if you have other fitness questions, we can help. We have a fitness expert who can answer your questions, and she'll be happy to offer you guidance on anything to do with the subject of fitness. If you're not a club person, you might be more interested in a home gym. Pat and her husband buy each other pieces of home gym equipment for their birthdays each year instead of purchasing other birthday gifts. As a result, when winter comes and it's tough to be outside for long, they have a beautifully equipped home gym.

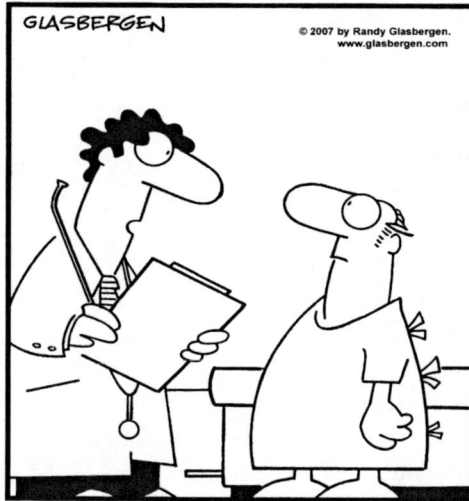

"The handle on your recliner does not count as an exercise machine."

You can do the same thing. If you want to get started, we mentioned the exercise mat as a good first step. In addition, we recommend a treadmill, a workbench with free weights, and an exercise ball. Mix in a DVD player and some really good exercise videos, and you've got everything you need to take your core strength and overall level of fitness to the next level.

Finally, we want to spend a moment talking about posture and how it relates to your core fitness and the health of your bone structure. You don't have to have military, ramrod-straight posture to be respected and admired in the workplace, but we all like people who stand tall. When people have good posture, they are signaling to the world that they respect themselves. That's a great message to send to people in the workplace and at home. Poor posture, by contrast, sends a negative message about who you are and how you feel about yourself. Physiologically, it's hard to stay happy when you're bent over! And if you've ever seen an older person who is bent over because of poor posture habits earlier in life, it's a real reminder that now is the time to take posture seriously.

An effective way to work on your posture as well as working out 90 percent of your muscles is to add Nordic Pole walking to your walking routines. By using Nordic Poles you can also burn up to 46 percent more calories when you walk. And it's a fun exercise, whether it's by yourself or with a group. You can go to our site and learn more about Nordic Pole walking (and even get the poles). It is the fastest growing sport in Europe due to the health benefits and the community spirit it creates. We also like it because it takes pressure off your joints while making you stand up straight. It's truly a fabulous way to build your strength, improve your posture, and burn more calories. **In the diagnostic tool, you will be asked about your posture.**

There you have it—four little exercises that you can do in the comfort and privacy of your own home or hotel room that can have a transformative effect on your core fitness and overall physical strength … and one great addition to your walking routine, Nordic Pole walking, to improve your strength, posture, and calorie burn. You've already addressed your cardiovascular strength, your mental state, and your diet. Now it's time to take the next step. Count on those four exercises to make a considerable difference in your life. Take it to the next level and hit the gym or create a home gym for yourself. Get your Nordic walking poles. But whatever you do, remember that the stronger you are, the greater your energy level will be and the more meaningful your life will be, at home and at work. Just adding a simple exercise to your daily routine, like doing squats while you brush your teeth, can make a significant difference in your wellness. And isn't that what really counts?

> *Remember that the stronger you are, the greater your energy level will be and the more meaningful your life will be, at home and at work.*

Online Diagnostic Tool Input:

Baseline repetitions of
Squats:_____
Crunches:_____
Leg Lifts:_____
Push-ups:_____
How is your posture?_____

Online Tracking Tools and Dashboard Input:

Strength ideas from this chapter to consider for the STAR™ process:

_____sets of _____reps of squats
_____sets of _____reps of leg lifts
_____sets of _____reps of crunches
_____sets of _____reps of push-ups
Doing thirty minutes of flexibility exercises such as yoga three days a week.
Attending an exercise class three times a week.
Walking with Nordic Poles three days a week.
Others:

_____

_____

☆   ☆   ☆

Please go to WalkStyles.com to input the above.

Chapter 6:
I Count on the People in My Life

Daily Step # 6: Walk 20 minutes with someone I love (family, friend or pet.)
Process: Use STAR™ and find people who support my healthy lifestyle and
walk with them at least 3 times per week.
Healthy lifestyle goal: Have meaningful relationships for the rest of my life.

Everything's harder when you go it alone. Everything's more fun, including getting in your steps, when you go with a buddy—whether it's a neighbor in the morning, a coworker at lunchtime, or a family member in the evening. When you plan to walk with others, it's easier and much more enjoyable to reach the goal of 10,000 steps a day. In this chapter, we'll talk about how to find walking partners and how to integrate the 10,000-steps concept into your already busy life.

In our society, we talk a lot about *activities*—going to the movies, watching the hot new show on TV, going out to eat, going for a drive, going to a show or a concert, or maybe stopping by the frozen yogurt stand or the ice cream store for dessert. But are these really activities? We should call them *passivities*! That's because each of these common behaviors requires us to be passive, not active. The most common ways that we entertain ourselves in our society mostly involve ... sitting down. Contrary to what you may have seen on the infomercials, it's awfully tough to lose weight, gain energy, or look your best while sitting in a chair! So the question is this: How do we find activities to replace the passivities that make up so much of our day?

Find more people with whom you can walk, and turn more things that you already do into active events instead of passive or sedentary ones.

We'd like to propose two approaches: find more people with whom you can walk, and turn more things that you already do into active events instead of passive or sedentary ones.

Let's take a moment and examine our current relationships. A startling study in the *New England Journal of Medicine*, one of the most highly regarded medical journals in the world, revealed the shocking truth that *friends help friends stay fat*.[17] The study's authors discovered that people who have poor eating habits tend to influence the eating decisions of others in their circle. Ever gone out to a restaurant with the intention of just having a salad or fish or some other healthy choice, and all of a sudden your best friend is imploring, "Come on, let's get some appetizers!" or "Let's just order a dessert for the table"? Then there's that age-old line that gets 'em every time: "What if I order it and everybody has some?"

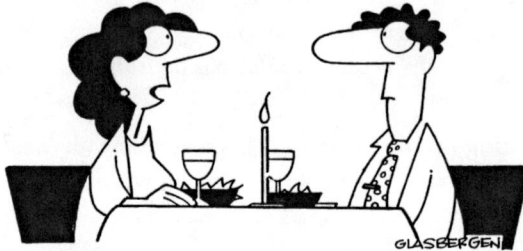

"I belong to a weight loss support group. We meet once a week and talk each other out of dieting."

Why do people bring others into their unhealthy eating habits? We're not psychologists, but we understand that it's easier to do something naughty if you can get someone else to do it with you. Most of us wish we could snap our fingers and magically take off those five, ten, fifteen, or more excess pounds, but somehow we just never get around to starting that diet. Or maybe we start it and have a hard time sticking to it. As a result, sometimes people feel guilty about not eating the way they know they should. They can somehow justify it to themselves more easily if they involve their friends in the same eating behavior. So those seemingly harmless questions of "Why don't we just order some appetizers?" or "What if I order it, and anybody who wants to can take some?" are actually more dangerous to our health than we realize. Our friends really *can* get us fat.

☆　　☆　　☆

Lynn's friends have never criticized each other for their weight gain. However, when she started adding steps, cutting down on the coffee drinks, and walking during one of her breaks, Lynn's friends asked her for ideas on how they can also start to lead healthier lifestyles. They noticed her newfound confidence and discipline. Andrea also noticed that Lynn had made some positive changes in her life and stopped by her desk to give her some recognition and encourage her to keep up the great work!

When Joe and his friends went out to eat, they'd order a bunch of appetizers, full dinners, and a couple of desserts "for the table." The table got to eat little of the dessert, though—they always seemed to stop in front of Joe. However, Joe has started to enjoy just a bite here or there knowing he is going to enter the food in his online food diary.

Andrea looks for the healthiest delicious item on the menu, enjoys a bite of a great appetizer, doesn't eat unrequested food (bread and butter, for example), and seldom eats dessert (okay, she savors a piece of dark chocolate almost every night …). Andrea wants to enjoy the conversation of her friends and family, so she fully engages in that part of a dinner out. In addition, she really wants to have the energy and strength to run her company and be a great parent, spouse, and friend.

☆   ☆   ☆

It's really amazing how many experiences and traditions in our society revolve around food. Birthday parties. Dinner parties. Thanksgiving and Christmas. Popcorn at the movies. Hot dogs, soda, beer, and ice cream at the ballpark. While food is a great way to bring people together, it's not the only way. We'd like to suggest that you create new traditions for your family that don't involve sitting and eating. For example, what about creating a family tradition of taking a walk together after Thanksgiving dinner? Or taking a family walk after dinner each evening? Or maybe taking a nice walk, instead of a big meal, after religious services? Or it could be as simple as taking a walk to the yogurt place instead of driving there.

Ask yourself how many supporters you have in your life. Any saboteurs? If so, why do you keep them around? Or why do you stay around them? Do the people in your world set goals? Do you know what those goals are? **In the diagnostic tool, you will be asked if your friends and family are supportive of you making healthy lifestyles changes and if you have at least one person in your life who offers you trustworthy advice about basic health matters.**

The key with your family, friends, and co-workers is to start weaving in activities that don't seem too overwhelming. If you try to put your family and friends on a forced march right off the bat, they're going to resist. But who could resist the idea of just taking one short walk? So invite your family, friends, and coworkers to join you in your quest for 10,000 steps each day. You'll be making your life easier … and their lives healthier. And if you do this at work, before long they just might name you CFO: Chief Fitness Officer!

It's possible that your friends will refuse to walk with you. They might whine and make excuses as to why they don't want to participate in your journey. Maybe they'll even be annoyed that you're suddenly expressing a new interest in being fit while they're still content being average. So the question then becomes: How do you find people who are also committed to making this change in their life and want to get out there and walk?

In our society today, it can be a challenge to find like-minded people. It can be a challenge just to find anyone—most of us today don't know our neighbors. If we don't have children in school, we might not know a single person on our block. Additionally, in our incredibly mobile society, people are always moving—for work-related reasons, for their retirement, to escape bad weather, or simply to try something new. As a result, most of us are much less rooted to our communities than we might have been a generation or two ago. In today's world, finding a real sense of community isn't easy.

We're here to help. One of the most popular features on WalkStyles.com is the database that gives you the opportunity to find fellow walkers, hikers, and joggers who live close to you, who move at your pace, and who want to exercise at the time of day that's convenient for you. There are so many new friends out there for us to meet when we decide to move from passivities to activities, and we want to help you meet them!

Let's talk now about the power that can be found in getting together with others—family members, new friends, old friends, and co-workers—to get in our steps.

The Power of the Group

We understand that it's tough to roll out of bed twenty minutes earlier than usual, especially if the temperature is on the chilly side, just to get in our steps. It's a lot easier to do it if you know your neighbor is waiting for you down the block. It's human nature not to want to let people down. Whether it's one person or a group, the power of planned walks with other people is enormous. It motivates us to get going and to get out of bed on those days when we'd rather just reach for the snooze button.

It's the same idea as the personal trainer at the gym. If you've got someone waiting for you, you're more likely to go. (Especially because you paid that person!) Here, you aren't paying your friends to walk with you. That's another advantage of walking—you don't need a trainer. You can just get together with your friends and go!

The Power of Fun

Quite frankly, once you get in with a walking group, you won't want to miss anything. You'll want to hear the latest episodes in everyone's lives, and the walk itself becomes a wonderful social time. Recently, Sue traveled to Iowa, where she met a woman whose mother had started a walking group more than fifty years earlier … and that group was still going strong. These women had first gotten together to walk when their children were in elementary school. It's no coincidence that all of these women survived into their eighties! Walking truly keeps us fit and young.

> *Walking truly keeps us fit and young.*

When we started WalkStyles, Inc., we wanted to find out how people could most easily incorporate 10,000 steps a day into their lives, so we held a focus group in Orange County. The idea was to get together for three months. Three years later, the Orange County walking group is stronger than ever. It's all about the power of community—just one of the many wonderful things about the process of taking steps to take control of your health and your fitness.

The Power of Family

Have you ever noticed that even families who eat dinner together (itself an increasingly rare phenomenon) quickly disperse, each to his or her own computer or TV screen? Dad's downstairs watching a game. Mom's in another room getting things done while watching the Discovery Channel®. The kids are supposed to be doing their homework, but they're in their rooms going on MySpace® or surfing the Net.

Technology is great, and we love the entertainment and education choices it offers. But when everybody's nestled in front of his or her own computer screen, it's hard for the idea of "family" to really take hold. So we recommend having "family meetings" while walking, perhaps after dinner. This is a great time for everybody to get together and share what happened in the course of their day, talk about what else is coming up on the calendar, or simply air out any issues that need discussion. It's a great way to make sure that your family is literally and figuratively headed in the right direction … and headed that way together!

The Power of Creativity

It's fun to create enjoyable opportunities that allow you to get your steps in. You can go to the mall and get steps, or you can go to the fair or the amusement park. All of these things are situations that don't involve sitting around—in a car, at the movies, or in a restaurant. You don't have to get every one of your 10,000 steps through walking! Dancing, cycling, swimming … any kind of movement counts. You can find a lot of creative ways to make your 10,000 steps. And didn't somebody once say that variety is the spice of life?

> *You don't have to get every one of your 10,000 steps through walking! Dancing, cycling, swimming…any kind of movement counts.*

The Power of Charity

It's great to sign up for charity walking events. You can join with your friends to raise money for worthwhile causes, and you can make new, like-minded friends at these events—people who are interested in staying healthy and in being involved. It's all about merging good works … with good walks!

The Power of Example

We really have to ask what kind of example we as a society are setting for our kids. Today, we are raising a generation of children prone to childhood obesity and forms of diabetes that only affected adults in the past. Because of sedentary lifestyles, computer games, and high-fat snack foods, our kids are heavier and less active than ever before.

It used to be that 50 percent of children walked to school, but today, sadly, that figure is closer to 10 percent.[18] The suggestion we'd like to offer here is to find ways to get your kids to walk to school. Instead of a carpool or the bus, you can arrange with other parents to create a walking group from your neighborhood to your children's school. You can use the free club tool at WalkStyles.com to set up a private club for the parents at your child's school. Set up a calendar designating which parents are leading the kids each day.

Perhaps you can take one day a week to walk with the group and find four other parents to do likewise. You'll get in your steps, and so will your kids. It's a powerful example of fitness and companionship for the next generation.

The Power of Healthy Choices

Here's another place where we can get really creative—think about the things you do now and ask yourself, "Is there a healthier way to do this? How can I do the same activity ... and still get in my steps?" For example, lots of people love to play golf. Why not get out of the cart and walk the course? Golfers will tell you that you get a much better "feel" for a course when you walk it. The pros walk, and it certainly doesn't hurt their game any! Obviously, there are some courses that do not lend themselves to walking. But why play those courses when you can find another one just as challenging that allows you to get out there and get in your steps?

Similarly, one of the things that guys like to do when they get together is to watch a game. The problem is that if you're going to be a good host, you've got to have the soda, beer, and munchies handy. But what if you and your friend went to the gym and watched the game from the vantage point of treadmills, stationary bikes, stair climbers, or other such equipment? In practically every gym, you can find big TVs mounted right over the fitness equipment for this very purpose. Why should the athletes on TV be the only ones getting any exercise on a Sunday afternoon? Watching the game is a perfect example of an activity that most people perform while sitting down (and munching out!). What other activities are there in your life that could be transformed into situations where you can get in your steps?

What activities are there in your life that could be transformed into situations where you can get in your steps?

The Power of Exploration

When most people take vacations and family trips, they spend a lot of time thinking about just relaxing and doing nothing. What could be better than sitting on the beach with a piña colada in your hand, watching the waves roll in? While we're all for balancing our frenetic lifestyles with a little bit of tropical R&R, we also highly recommend planning vacations around opportunities to get out and walk. Recently, Sue and her husband took their family to Chicago to explore the city, and they walked everywhere. That way, they were still able to enjoy the great food for which Chicago is famous … the deep-dish pizza, the steaks. But because they walked everywhere, they didn't take home a few excess pounds around their middles as "souvenirs" from the journey.

The Power of Accountability

Before we started our company, Sue was a typically stressed corporate leader, and Pat was an executive in the banking industry. Pat's own personal challenge was one with which many women can identify: weight gain after pregnancies. She didn't gain a tremendous amount of weight … but she had a tough time losing that weight each time after she gave birth. We lived in different cities, but every day we would e-mail each other our steps. It turned into a friendly competition to see who was finding the most intriguing and enjoyable ways to get in her steps, but it really wasn't about competition. Instead, we were holding each other accountable to our commitment to ourselves to get out there and walk. From personal experience and from the testimony of countless walkers we've met through our business, we deeply believe in the power of accountability. We all need a little support and shoring up from time to time. Finding another person to hold us accountable, and doing the same thing for that person, is a great way to reinforce our commitment to our steps.

In short, you can count on your friends, your family, and your coworkers who share your commitment and passion for bringing fitness into your life in the most enjoyable manner possible. So now is the time to be inspired to make not only your life better, but to inspire those around you to enjoy life, health, fitness, and a little bit of fresh air like never before. Remember, just spending twenty minutes walking with a friend will improve your life and theirs. You can count on others, and they can count on you!

Online Diagnostic Tool Input:

Are your family and friends supportive of you making healthy
lifestyle changes?
Is there at least one person in your life who provides trustworthy
advice about your health?

Online Tracking Tool and Dashboard Input:

Other relationship ideas from this chapter to consider for the STAR™
process:

Taking a twenty-minute walk with another person.
Walking my children to or from school two days a week.
Having a sit-down meal with my family and taking a walk afterwards
three days a week.
Others:

_____

_____

☆   ☆   ☆

Please go to WalkStyles.com to input the above.

Chapter 7:
I Count on My Workplace

Daily Step # 7: Take a 20 minute dedicated walk in my work day.
Process: Use STAR™ to arrange walking meetings and get more activity into my work day.
Healthy lifestyle goal: Be productive, engaged and successful for the rest of my life.

Most of us spend the majority of our waking hours at work, so it would be great if we could fit into our work schedules the concept of getting in our 10,000 steps. There is certainly a need for the stress-busting benefits of walking during the workday. Let's face it—people are working harder than ever. We're now working an average of forty-seven hours per week, and we're working harder to keep our jobs. Every time we pass by a gas station and see those prices climbing, we know that we're getting more and more squeezed financially. And, of course, there are those health care costs. It's a tough time to be an employee *or* an employer.

There's good news though, and, as you might have guessed, it all revolves around walking. The human body simply wasn't designed for all the hours of sitting. The body was designed to move! We need to learn how to be more active in our workplaces. And we also have to consider skyrocketing health care costs for employers. Obesity alone raises the average employer's health costs $285,000 a year for every 1,000 employees.[19]

According to the U.S. Department of Health and Human Services, for every 100 employees in this country:[20]

- 27 have cardiovascular disease
- 24 have high blood pressure
- 50 or more have high cholesterol
- 26 are overweight by 20 percent or more
- 10 are heavy drinkers
- 59 don't get adequate exercise
- 44 suffer from stress

Yikes! A workforce that doesn't take care of itself ends up costing much more in health care, because health problems inevitably arise. A company that starts a wellness program cares about its workers and also positively affects the financial health of the company. The good news is that a walking program can directly help with all but the heavy drinking. And indirectly, with the new healthy attitude that comes from making your step count and using the STAR™ process, the drinking could decrease as well. The message is that we all need to do our part—employers need to offer wellness programs and employees need to use them!

Companies that focus on wellness can use the health care dollars they save to reduce the cost of their products, do more marketing and advertising, hire more people, and pay more to the people they employ. There is a direct correlation between a company's bottom line and the employees' waistlines. If we aren't taking care of our own health, we're not the only ones who suffer. So do our fellow employees, because our health care costs are taking dollars out of the company … and out of their pockets. At WalkStyles.com, we have lots of data to share with you about the need and the effectiveness of having a corporate wellness program.

✶　　✶　　✶

Our CEO friend Andrea has already implemented a terrific wellness program, including a walking program. She also is a good role model and parks far from the office door, takes steps versus the elevator, and while waiting for her flights, is seen walking the airport while talking on her phone. In the company walking contest, everyone wants Andrea on their team for a good reason! The incentive program she put in place for most steps per team offers choices of time off, reduction in health care costs, or attractive workout clothing and is creating a fun, but healthy competition around the company. Joe is enrolled in the wellness program at work and his team is using the ideas in the articles on walking and wellness on WalkStyles.com to increase their daily activity. These suggestions are helping his team consistently score high numbers in their daily step count. He is also determined to get his waistline below 40 inches and is beginning to see progess. Lynn's recent health scare was a wake-up call, and her daily walks and eliminating the calorie-loaded coffee drinks have not only made her popular with her walking team, but have resulted in her first true weight loss in years. She is feeling better about herself and has become a much more enthusiastic and fun person to be around.

✶　　✶　　✶

In the diagnostic tool, you will be asked if your company has a wellness plan and, if so, do you participate.

There's more good news—it might actually be easier to find people at work with whom you can walk than it is at home. Your family members may be stuck in their sedentary ways (at least for now!). But in the workplace, you're likely to find a broader range of attitudes toward exercise. Chances are, there's someone in your area or department who would be delighted to get up and walk with you for twenty minutes during the lunch break, or at other times of the day. You truly can count on your coworkers, and they can count on you—for motivation, for inspiration, and for developing habits that revolve around fitness instead of the way so many of us actually live today.

> *You truly can count on your coworkers, and they can count on you—for motivation, for inspiration, and for developing habits that revolve around fitness instead of the way so many of us actually live today.*

Stress Buster

Walking is a wonderful stress buster. Even on a good day at work, we're still sitting at our desks or work stations, usually hunched over our computers for hours at a time. Our bodies literally don't get a break! They need to stretch and move around, and walking is a great way to relieve the tension that comes from just sitting and working. We're rough enough on our bodies on a good day; more often than not, a lot of our workdays are extremely stressful. Walking provides the perfect solution. There's really nothing like a good twenty-minute walk to let go of the tension that comes from deadlines, bosses, expectations, ringing phones, e-mail inboxes filled to overflowing, and all the other demands of the typical workday. Getting away from our desks and into the fresh air is the greatest thing in the world for the over-stressed, over-worked man or woman.

Problem Solving

Another great thing to do while you're out walking is to focus on a work problem you want to solve. We've discovered that solutions to even the most complicated work problems come much more quickly and easily in sunshine than under fluorescent lights back at the office. One twenty-minute walk can provide you with the idea of a lifetime ... or at least the idea you've been looking for in order to solve a problem that's been bugging you all day.

> *One twenty-minute walk can provide you with the idea of a lifetime.*

When we started WalkStyles, Inc., we were trying to figure out how to name one of our signature products, a device that lets you measure your steps. Sue, Pat, and Dina were all out walking together, trying to solve this problem and come up with a great name. Sue wanted to create a personal dashboard, similar to the dashboard she used in corporate America for business metrics, so she was toying with the word dash for their new fitness monitor. Dina remembered a poem she had seen on the Internet by a woman named Linda Ellis. The poem talked about how we have a date of birth and a date of death and a dash that separates the two, and the dash symbolizes or encapsulates our entire life. Suddenly, all three got chills as they realized that DashTrak® covered not only the hard metric side of making a goal, but also the spiritual benefits of being more active. And that's how we came up with the name DashTrak® … while walking!

You might have noticed that here we had *three* people walking together trying to solve a work problem. Walking can have great benefits for groups solving problems together. A typical group meeting is structured around a conference table, and the group dynamics are dictated by the fact that people are, for the most part, looking each other in the eye. It's hard to bring up a new idea under those circumstances. We can be afraid to share an idea because other people might look at us with an expression that says, "What on earth are you thinking? That's crazy! That could never work!" By contrast, when people are out walking together instead of seated around a table, they can have ideas and blurt them out, secure in the knowledge that no one's going to be looking them in the eye and saying, "That's crazy!" That's why we say that ideas flourish in sunlight. So the next time your group has a problem to solve, tell them all to hit the road. (Be careful about telling your boss to hit the road. We don't want you to get into any trouble!)

Conflict Resolution

Another great thing we can do while walking is to take the strain out of a personal relationship. Let's say we have angry words with a coworker, a boss, or a loved one. Before we make a bad situation worse, it's always a great idea to just step away, calm down, and come back to ourselves. Twenty minutes of walking goes a long way toward letting tempers cool off and allowing tensions to dissolve. And remember: you can never get in trouble for what you *don't* say! So another great use of solitary walk breaks is the opportunity they afford to soften disagreements with the important people in our lives, whether it's at home or at work.

Many of our client companies have adopted the policy of resolving disputes through the process of taking brief walks—somehow walking provides the wonderful benefit of clearing the air between two people who are having a dispute over one issue or another. It's hard to walk with someone and still stay upset, because walking is such a social activity. There's nothing like hitting the road to find some common ground!

One-on-Ones

You don't need an entire group to have a great meeting at work. We encourage supervisors to take their staff members out for one-on-one walks to discuss issues in the workplace in an atmosphere that is more conducive to privacy and creativity. The next time you have a meeting scheduled with a team member, why not take that meeting outside? Why not invite your coworker to join you for a quick hike around the building or factory or plant? If the weather is inclement, there's often a nearby mall you can duck into. As a result, you'll both get some much-needed exercise, and we have no doubt that you'll be seeing your workplace problems and opportunities in a whole new light. For tips on effective walking meetings, please go to WalkStyles.com.

One Good Thing ...

If you are a manager, you'll want to introduce walking breaks, walking meetings, walking one-on-ones, and walking group discussions into your workplace with enthusiasm and authenticity. We've found that once one or two people start walking regularly, others become curious and get involved as well. Before you know it, the entire department is going out for some much-needed walks, and everybody's happier.

Another benefit of adding walking to the workplace is that people tend to become a bit more health-conscious in general. Consider the typical office potluck. Nobody has time to prepare a healthy meal for such an event. In most offices, even if someone took the time and trouble to make one, the healthy dish would likely go untouched. The most successful items from a popularity point of view include those infamous calorie-laden eight-layer bean dips and similar dishes that take little time to prepare (and lots of time to work off the calories they contain).

> *Another benefit of adding walking to the workplace is that people tend to become a bit more health-conscious in general.*

We've discussed in earlier chapters the fact that once we start walking, we start thinking more and more about other aspects of our lifestyles, including how, what, and when we eat. If you're starting to shed some unwanted pounds because you're out there getting your steps in, it's a little less beguiling to sit there in front of the computer screen at work just munching on whatever snack food is at hand. When people start walking in the workplace, those eight-layer bean dips gradually give way to better choices—maybe even healthy salads. And then people actually start eating those salads. It really happens! So when you acculturate your team members and coworkers to the idea of walking, they generally step up the quality of their eating habits as well.

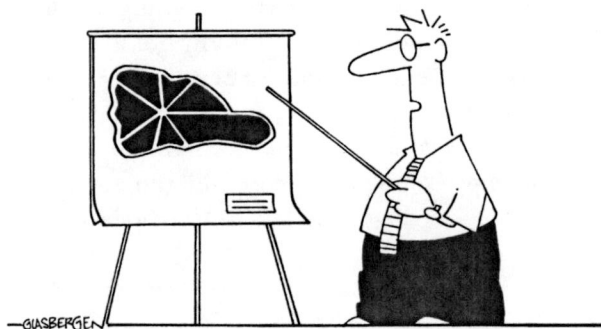

"At the request of those who are following a low-carb diet, my pie chart has been replaced by a steak chart."

Walking the Walk Counts

Those of us who work in offices and cubicles are not the only people who ought to be getting out and walking. The CEO and the board of companies need to be getting out there as well and getting in their steps. In many companies, occasional board meetings are held in luxurious five-star hotels or conference centers. All well and good, but why not conduct board meetings onsite, and have the C-level executives and board members actually get out and walk the floors of the office buildings and factories where the actual work of the company gets done? When the boss is walking, it sets a great example about fitness for the rest of the organization. And it means an enormous amount when top executives and board members actually meet line workers, ask them what they do, ask them what could be better, and so on. There's even a term for it—MBWA, or Management By Walking Around. Many of America's most successful executives do this, and we think everybody should!

Team Building

What about days off? In practically every city and town today, you can find charity walks that benefit local charitable organizations or national health foundations. A great team-building exercise (that actually allows people to get in some exercise) is to get involved in these charity walks. If the walks are long, then team members can plan on getting together for training walks. This is an opportunity that works to the advantage of all concerned— the employees get a chance to do something for themselves, and the company as a whole gets a chance to support something important in the community. Both of us have organized groups of walkers and raised thousands of dollars on charity walks. We also get to meet new people, reach our daily step goal, and have fun!

Engage the Extended Team

Back at the office, there are some people you can take for a walk … and they'll have to go, whether they want to or not. Those are your vendors and suppliers. Sue says she always takes her vendors and suppliers out for walks—if they want her business, they can't say no! You've got a captive audience and an instant partner every time a vendor or salesperson drops in. So that's another great way to get some steps in during the working day.

The great thing about walking with others from your office, whether they are coworkers, managers, or people who report to you, is that everybody comes back just a little bit friendlier, a little bit more relaxed, and a little bit more casual after having walked together. It's not just an opportunity to get in our steps and feel better about ourselves. It's about developing stronger bonds and ties in the workplace, which really does increase morale and productivity.

> *Walking with coworkers isn't just an opportunity to get in our steps and feel better about ourselves. It's about developing stronger bonds and ties in the workplace.*

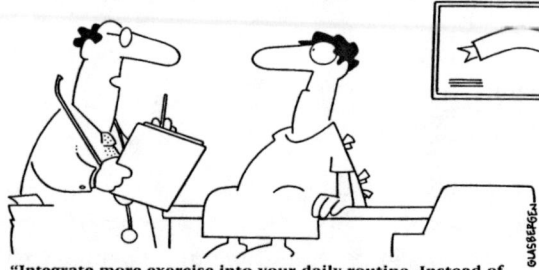

Copyright 2003 by Randy Glasbergen.
www.glasbergen.com

"Integrate more exercise into your daily routine. Instead of taking the elevator, climb up the side of the building. When you pass a coworker in the hall, insist on a game of leap-frog. Use kick boxing to post messages on your bulletin board. Stir your coffee with your toes. Arm wrestle your clients..."

Your Company Goes "Green" Too

As we mentioned in an earlier chapter, we live in a time of great concern for the environment and walking is about as "green" an activity as you can find—it's as good for the planet as it is for the walker. It doesn't trigger greenhouse gasses or threaten the ozone layer. When we walk it gets us out of our cars, which means we're using less fossil fuel and ever so slightly reducing our dependence on foreign oil producers. Walking isn't just good personal policy; it's a great planet policy as well. And when you go green with your exercise program, it means fewer trips to the gas station ... which leaves more green in your wallet or purse!

The *Washington Post* recently published a report that said if all Americans from ten to seventy-four drove thirty minutes a day less and walked thirty minutes a day more, it would curb the annual U.S. emissions of carbon dioxide by sixty-four million tons, would save six and a half billion gallons of gas, and would eliminate three billion pounds from our waistlines.[22] The workplace is as great a place as any to create a culture of walking and fitness. Workers of the world, unite! You've got nothing to lose but some stress, a few unwanted pounds, and those unhealthy snacks. First one to the stairs wins!

Be More Productive

Finally, exercise is good for the brain. Want to be more productive? Exercise your body *and* your mind. Solving complex problems at work, reading textbooks or similarly involved articles, and doing crossword puzzles, Sudoku, or any other kind of brain-strengthening game will make you more alert and productive. However, just physically exercising is keeping your brain younger.

Did you know that about one third of the working population forgets about deadlines or important work information? Exercise helps, physically *and* mentally. When you get in your steps, you'll be more on the ball and ready to tackle all the unique challenges your job presents.

☆　　☆　　☆

Find ways to make walking a part of every workday. Whether it's your boss, coworkers, or employees, others will take notice. So even when you're at work, work it … and work it good. Andrea sets a great example for her team. Joe noticed increased productivity gains. And Lynn has delivered her last three projects ahead of time! Andrea is making sure they are rewarded for their efforts.

☆　　☆　　☆

Remember, just making one change in your workday, such as always taking twenty minutes at lunch to walk, will pay big dividends in your health and with your productivity. So it's time to Set, Track, Achieve, and Reward your progress as we count on the workplace to help us develop our healthy "workstyles."

Online Diagnostic Tool Input:

Does your company have a wellness plan, and if so, do you participate?

Online Tracking Tools and Dashboard Input:

Workplace ideas from this chapter to consider for the STAR™ process:

Taking a twenty-minute walk on my lunchbreak each day.
Taking a fifteen-minute walk break in the morning each day.
Taking a fifteen-minute walk break in the afternoon each day.
Delivering five messages in person rather than by email each day.
Parking one thousand feet away from the office door each day.
Conducting two one-on-one meetings while walking each day.
Others:

_____

_____

★ ★ ★

Please go to WalkStyles.com to input the above.

Chapter 8:
I Count My Blessings

Daily Step #8: Walk 20 minutes alone.
Process: Use STAR™ to find the time just for me, to journal and to note at least 5 things I am thankful for each day.
Healthy lifestyle goal: Be positive and thankful for the rest of my life.

When you think about it, there are very few times in the course of a day when we are left to our own thoughts. Most people choose to wake up to an alarm clock playing music, news, or even idle chitchat—anything besides that nasty buzzing sound. So we're subjected to other people's thoughts and ideas from the very moment we wake up.

Then, as we start our day, our companion as we get ready and grab breakfast is the TV. If we commute to work in the car, we usually have the car radio on or we are talking on the phone. Not too many people drive to work in a quiet car! If we happen to be taking public transportation, we're probably listening to music or some kind of download on an iPod® or, for the really old-school, our Walkman®. When we get to work, we're generally thinking about work (at least *some* of the time) and not our own lives. And so it goes through the commute home, dinner (often with the TV on), a few hours of sitcoms or dramas or reality shows, and then off to bed.

So much of what we hear is negative. People complain about everything. The news is depressing. All that negativity has a powerful effect on our psyche. It's tough sometimes to be positive in such a negative world. How's your outlook? Can you see the positive side of things?

Over the course of the typical day, we hear a lot of voices. But the only voice we seldom hear is our own. In this chapter, we'd like to suggest that if you miss out on yourself as a conversation partner when you're walking, you're missing out on the best conversation of all. Spending more time by yourself will make you more productive in all areas of your life.

If you miss out on yourself as a conversation partner when you're walking, you're missing out on the best conversation of all.

Relax and energize

Most of us live in a very stressful state of mind. One great way to shake off the stress of work, family, or even world events, is to enjoy a twenty minute or more walk alone. This is your chance to decompress and put everything in perspective. Develop a rhythm with your arms and feet. You'll find yourself releasing the tensions of the day.

If you pick up the pace, you will find the endorphins kicking in and you can transcend the daily grind. Exercise is truly amazing for the ability to reduce your anxiety as well as to lift your spirits. It is the perfect tonic for your busy day. **In the diagnostic tool you'll be asked if you spend time on yourself.**

Escape

If you want to truly remove yourself, put on your headset and walk listening to your favorite music. You'll develop a faster pace and will probably go longer with this wonderful way to tune out the rest of the world. Just remember, that when walking outside with a headset, be very aware of traffic, signals and other potential hazards.

Gain Perspective

Another reason to walk by ourselves is to appreciate nature. It is important to realize that there is more to the world than *you*. By recognizing that we all play a role in the larger scheme, we are able to reduce stress, gain perspective, and become energized and more productive. Often, until we start walking

> *Walking by ourselves gives us a great chance to stop and smell the flowers…literally.*

regularly, we don't realize just how much beauty there is in the neighborhood, city, or region where we reside. Just about every city or town has beautiful parks, walking trails, beaches, or other attractive places for walking. We could go our whole lives without ever recognizing the beauty that surrounds us. Getting out and walking puts us in touch with nature, especially with the four seasons.

Pat likes to say that when she walks down the same streets over the course of the year, she gets to see fresh snow, the new buds of spring, the green leaves of summer, and the falling leaves of autumn. In our culture, we are so technology-minded that we tend to forget the natural world that surrounds us. We rely not so much on nature, but on man-made things to get us everything we need, from our cell phones and PDAs to our computers and our cars. When we walk with others, we're more likely to focus on the conversation and not even notice the scenery. Walking by ourselves gives us a great chance to stop and smell the flowers … literally.

Learn Something

What if the weather is bad? Head for the mall, or jump on a treadmill at home or at the gym. But if you do so, think about using at least one of your twenty-minute breaks to learn something new. Our muscles need stretching … and so do our minds. If you have an iPod™ or something similar, you can program it with inspirational material and self-help books. Or how about buying an audiotape or MP3 download of *War and Peace*? With enough twenty-minute walk breaks, you might actually be able to finish it and have one of the world's greatest pieces of literature under your belt. You can even use your walking time to learn a new language—there's no limit to how you can expand your mind.

> *Walking by yourself gives you a great opportunity to get back in touch with who you are and where your life is going.*

Just one great idea can increase your income, your happiness, the quality of your relationships, your health and fitness … there's no limit to what you can learn if you keep your ears open. Whether you're walking inside or outside, walking by yourself gives you a great opportunity to get back in touch with who you are and where your life is going.

Have a Plan

It's also great to attach a goal to some of the walks you take. One of Pat's goals was to walk through every forest preserve in her city over the course of a year. She was amazed at the beauty, the animals, and the peace that she experienced on these walks. When she achieved her goal, she not only experienced a great sense of satisfaction but had managed to see some of her city's most beautiful secret treasures too.

Sue set a goal to help spread the word about the power of community and wellness and went to all fifty state capitals in fifty weeks and led 10,000-step (of course!) walks through each of these inspiring cities. The WalkStyles

WeWhoWalk™ tour was an amazing journey, and you can walk these walks by going to WalkStyles.com and downloading each of these maps.

Ask Questions

What else can we do with our minds in order to maximize the value of our walks? We can ask ourselves better questions. Maxwell Maltz, in his groundbreaking book *Psycho Cybernetics*, wrote that the human brain is a computer, but not just any kind of computer—it's a "question-answering machine." According to Maltz, whenever we ask ourselves a question, the brain thinks and thinks and thinks until it comes up with a really great answer to that question. Unfortunately, most of us use this power in a negative way. We ask ourselves things like, "Why did I mess up that situation at work?"

And the brain thinks and thinks and thinks … until it comes to the conclusion that we're just not very smart! Maltz says that if we want to have a better life, we need to ask ourselves better questions. So here are some good questions that we'd like you to ask yourself as you walk:

"What can I do today to make this a great day for myself and those around me?"

"What can I do for others today?"

Think About Others

While you are walking you may want to think about the special people in your life. A friend of Pat's would put a blank card on his desk every day before leaving work. The next morning he writes a special message on it to a friend or family member and sends it along with an article he's clipped from the paper. He uses his early morning walk time to think about those people who are meaningful in his life but whom he hasn't contacted in a while and then follows through with these special notes.

If you tell your subconscious that good things are happening, it's going to believe you.

84

Appreciate

"What am I grateful for?" So often, we fail to count our blessings, and we focus only on the negative in our lives. If all we think about is ill health, failing relationships, problems at work, and money troubles, we end up getting more of the same. One theory we have heard that may explain this is that we use only 5 percent of our brain when we think on a conscious level, and the 95 percent of the brain that represents the unconscious mind cannot distinguish between reality and whatever the 5 percent conscious part of our brain *says* is reality. In other words, your subconscious cannot distinguish between what's really happening and what you *say* is really happening. So if you tell your subconscious that good things are happening, it's going to believe you! And the easiest way to get yourself into a great frame of mind is to think about all the wonderful things that are already happening in your life right now.

Unfortunately, most of us spend way too much time thinking about what we don't have instead of what we do have. But what if we were to take time and consciously make lists of all the things we are grateful for right now? We could start with our health and our physical bodies. We could think about how grateful we are for each of the senses that we have—our ability to hear, to taste, to see, to feel, and to smell. It sounds a little corny, but when you think about what a miracle each of those gifts represents, it definitely gets us thinking about how remarkable and wonderful we are ... whether or not we've been able to lose those last five (or ten, or fifteen, or more!) pounds. So often we focus on what's wrong with our bodies instead of what's right with them. What if, instead of focusing on the negative while we were out there walking, we concentrated on the many reasons we have to be grateful just for our physical selves? **In the diagnostic tool, you will be asked if you are able to identify five different things you are truly grateful for in your life.**

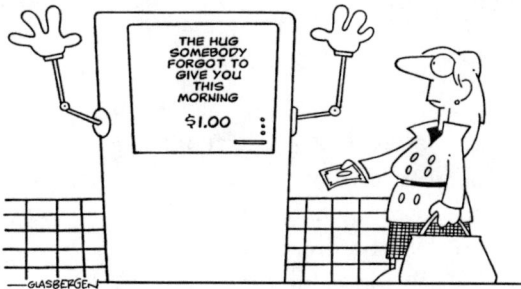

Journal

It is a good time to mention how important journaling is to helping you understand how you are achieving your healthy goals. Journaling allows you to capture the thoughts you have had while walking and gives you a record to go back and review your days. It is so powerful. You can journal online at WalkStyles.com, use our spiral-bound book, or use another. We encourage you to capture your memories. If you take the time each day to enter those five things you are grateful for, you'll truly start focusing on the positive aspects of your life. Think of the time you will save by not wasting valuable moments dwelling on the negative.

☆　　☆　　☆

How do Lynn, Joe, and Andrea think about their lives? That's easy: Andrea makes things happen. Andrea has carried a personal/professional goal list since high school days, updating and revising it as goals were met. She uses a dashboard at work for her company's daily metrics and uses her personal dashboard to make sure she is taking good care of herself. Her family regularly conducts family meetings and talks about what they want to accomplish, such as vacations, major holidays, celebrations, community service, college planning, etc. Each person in the family has realized the value of planning and taking responsibility for certain behaviors or tasks that might be required of them. Joe wants what Andrea has been able to achieve, but he has never before clearly articulated or written down any goals or obstacles that could get in the way of achieving them. Therefore, it has taken so much longer for anything desired to happen, and when it does, it many times comes as a surprise. He has begun using a dashboard to measure his personal daily goals and feels more in control of his health. And then we have Lynn, who has begun to realize that she would no longer tolerate life just passing her by and has started setting up small, daily goals she is determined to achieve.

☆　　☆　　☆

Author and motivator Zig Ziglar likes to tell his seminar audiences that he wishes he could sell them each their own brains … for $100,000 per person. He says everybody would be happier. Everybody would value their brains more, because they had paid so much for them,

> *The more you think about what you're grateful for, the happier you'll be.*

and he would be happy too, because he would collect $100,000 from so many people! But why not take a moment and be grateful for our marvelous brains *without* having to shell out a hundred thousand bucks? Our brains that have such amazing capacities to think, to create, to experience, to feel, and to love. They call the brain "the three-pound universe" because it's a computer that weighs only three pounds and yet will never be matched, not even by the greatest works of humanity.

Chances are, if you're reading this, you've got a place to sleep and you've got clothing—and maybe pretty nice clothing at that. You've got money in your pocket, food in the refrigerator, probably a car in the driveway ... okay, maybe it's not your dream car, but it is yours. So don't let the advertising culture that surrounds us give you a feeling of dissatisfaction with what you have and how you look. Instead, the more you think about what you're grateful for, the happier you'll be. And there's nothing like the combination of physical movement through walking and developing your mental attitude of gratitude to make you feel like a million bucks.

The Future

The final suggestion we'd like to offer has to do with thinking about where our lives are headed. Again, when most of us think about the future, we tend to view it with anxiety and fear. What if I lose my job? What if my car breaks down? What if he (or she) leaves me?

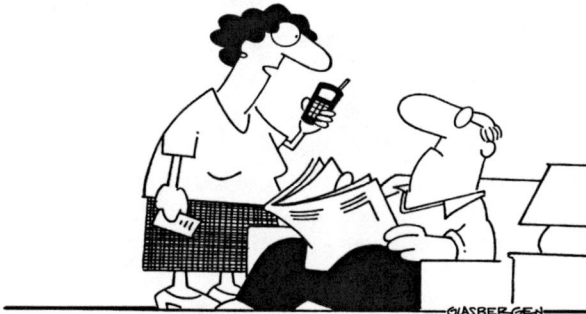

Copyright 2004 by Randy Glasbergen.
www.glasbergen.com

"Good news — they found you a donor for a smile transplant!"

We understand that all these fears may be entirely legitimate. But worrying takes valuable time out of our lives and many of us lose sleep over it. What if we envisioned a future in positive terms instead? Here's a suggestion: Imagine that you are addressing a group of people three months from today. Who they are or why they've gathered together to listen to you isn't important. But as you walk, pretend that you are making a speech to them about how all the problems that you were worried about have been resolved. Let's pretend that today is February 1. So in your imaginary speech, it's May 1. Your speech might go something like this:

"Today is May 1, and I'm very excited that you've joined me for my talk. I'm happy to tell you that all the things I was worried about three months ago worked out so beautifully that I can't even believe it. The challenge I was having at work led to a breakthrough, and that turned into a promotion and a big raise. In fact, I won the sales competition, and I'll be going on a cruise in the Caribbean next month! On top of that, the issues that I had in my relationship have been completely resolved, and the two of us are doing better than ever. Our kids are doing great, and we've decided to buy a new car. And that health scare I had three months ago—it turned out to be nothing at all."

Obviously you've got to tailor the speech to fit your own specific situation, and you don't want to make it so Pollyanna-ish that even you can't believe it. But the thing is, we're always imagining the future. So who says we have to imagine a less-than-perfect one? That's why it can be fun to get out there and address your imaginary group about all the success you will have achieved over the next three months—or whatever period of time you choose.

In sum, it's great to walk with family, friends, and coworkers. But if you leave out the person in the mirror, you'll be missing out on the greatest walking partner of them all—and that's you! Remember, just one small daily goal, such as journaling five minutes a day, can make a world of difference in the long run. So count your blessings, count your steps, Set, Track, Achieve, and Reward in a new level of connection, not just with everyone else in your life … but with you, yourself.

> *If you leave out the person in the mirror, you'll be missing out on the greatest walking partner of them all… and that's you!*

Online Diagnostic Tool Input:

Do you spend time on yourself?
Can you name five things you are grateful for?

Online Tracking Tools and Dashboard Input:

Blessing ideas from this chapter to consider for the STAR™ process:

Taking a twenty-minute walk alone each day.
Doing one random act of kindness each day.
Journaling for five minutes each day.
Meditating for five minutes each day.
Telling one person "I love you" each day.
Others:

_____

_____

☆   ☆   ☆

Please go to WalkStyles.com to input the above.

Chapter 9:
I Count on Myself

Daily Step # 9: Do my daily goals in 10 week increments.
Process: Use STAR™ to develop the discipline I need to reach my healthy lifestyle goals.
Healthy lifestyle goal: Make my healthy daily goals part of my lifestyle for the rest of my life.

Take a bow! If you've been making changes to your lifestyle while reading this book, you're either walking 10,000 steps a day or you're very close to reaching that mark. As a result, you've bonded more deeply with coworkers, friends, and loved ones. You've almost certainly lost weight because you're moving more and therefore burning up more calories. And you're probably eating better because, as we've discussed, it's psychologically harder to eat poorly when you know you've invested so much effort in getting your steps in.

What's happening at work? You're inevitably getting more done in less time and with a better attitude. Walking during lunch or on breaks is helping you become more alert, as well as giving you the opportunity to know coworkers on a whole new level. Perhaps you even had a walking coaching session with your boss last week, and the changes you've been making have not gone unnoticed!

And you're not just feeling stronger every day, you're actually *getting* stronger, because you've begun to work into your life some or all of the strength exercises we talked about in the previous chapter. You're just a lean, mean walking machine!

☆   ☆   ☆

Our friends Andrea, Joe, and Lynn have made great strides (no pun intended!) as well. Andrea is thrilled by the improved morale and productivity increases she is seeing as a result of the company's wellness program. And, even though she was in good shape before starting, Andrea has personally noticed that she has lost a percent of body fat due to the increased level of activity in the workplace.

By eating better and exercising, Joe dropped ten pounds and went from a forty-inch waist down to thirty-seven. He still isn't at his high school weight, but the crunches and jogging in place he does while watching football games are certainly paying off! He is feeling better about himself, as well as healthier, and is determined to keep at it. With his new goal setting skills, he has developed a plan with his boss to get him promotable in six months. He is so appreciative of the company for rewarding him personally and professionally.

Even Lynn is on the upswing—she replaced those coffee drinks with water and rarely misses walking each day. She is now up to 6,500 steps and has gotten to 10,000 on a number of days when she walked along the sidelines at soccer and baseball games or helped her children learn dance steps by practicing with them … (yes, dance steps count!). Although she still occasionally visits the dessert table, there has definitely been a change in the frequency of those trips. Lynn has more energy and is becoming a star employee as well as an inspiration for her children. She even has been researching online classes to complete her college degree. Lynn feels empowered for the first time in a long time, and she is finally rewarding herself for achieving her daily goals.

☆   ☆   ☆

The theme of this chapter is simple: Now that you've accomplished all these wonderful, healthy changes in your life, you need to sustain them and truly make them part of your lifestyle forever.

We like the idea of ten weeks to get a new healthy habit woven into your lifestyle. We have learned that it takes three weeks to build a habit, but if you use the STAR™ process over a ten-week period, you will own that habit. Even better, you will also see the bigger results of your new habit. If you did push-ups for ten weeks, you will start seeing the definition in your upper arms. A great reward for that may be a trip to the beach or new clothes or lifting your own luggage into the plane's overhead compartment!

> *We have learned that it takes three weeks to build a habit, but if you use this STAR™ process over a ten-week period, you will own that habit.*

Many people don't like to set goals, for a variety of different reasons. They may not believe they're capable of reaching their goals, and so they want to protect themselves from disappointment. Or they know it takes a certain amount of discipline and stick-to-it-ness to reach a goal, and it just sounds like too much work. That might have been your attitude before you started down the path toward 10,000 steps a day, but we suspect that if you ever thought that way in the past, you certainly no longer think that way now. You know there is power in setting simple, daily goals you can weave into your lifestyle. There's nothing like getting results to make us hungry for more success, more joy, better relationships, more money, and more of all the important things that money can't buy. So the question we'd like to pose to you right now is this: What would you like next in your life?

The best way to set your lifestyle goals is to think about a time in the not-too-distant future—say, one to three years from now—and ask yourself:

> *A dream is nothing more than a hope or a wish until you quantify it and track it—and then it becomes a goal.*

1. What do I want in my personal life?
2. What do I want in my work life?
3. What do I want in my financial life?
4. How do I serve the world?

Take a few moments and answer each of those questions in just a few words. Maybe in your work life you want to become a supervisor and increase your pay by 25 percent. Maybe in your personal life you want to be engaged to be married by one year from today. Maybe in your financial life you want to have a specific net worth or a specific amount of money in your retirement account. And in terms of serving the world, that's really up to you as well. Do you want to volunteer a certain amount of time with an organization you admire? Is there a certain amount of fundraising that you might like to do for a group? What would be the best way for you to give back, since you've been given so much? What is the footprint you want to leave as your legacy?

As we've seen, most successful people in the world recognize that setting their goals and tracking their actual results have enormous power. And a goal is not a goal if it doesn't include something to measure and the timetable for reaching the goal. Remember, those bigger lifestyle goals won't happen overnight. You can reach them by Setting, Tracking, Achieving, and Rewarding daily goals that will lead you to those bigger results.

It is all about moving forward. Never take your eye off your dashboard and your steps. Never take your health for granted, keep counting on yourself and keep moving forward. Let the STAR™ process guide you.

> *Never take your eye off your dashboard and your steps. Never take your health for granted. Keep counting on yourself and keep moving forward.*

Walking Goals

Since this book is about making your step count, perhaps some of your goals should include walking. It's time for some unlimited thinking about where walking can take you. How about planning a walking tour across the south of France? Or, what about taking part in a Susan G. Komen Race for the Cure™? People could be sponsoring you, and you could be raising significant amounts of money for an important charity.

You can be getting your family, friends, and coworkers involved, too. You can get them on the path to 10,000 steps, and you can get them involved with the charitable causes you've chosen. This way, you'll be helping them change their own lives and transform the world around them as well. You've made so many strides toward having a better life for yourself. Now you've got a responsibility to maintain the changes you've created and help others get to the same point.

We'd also like to suggest that you take *a walk on the wild side.* So far, everything we've discussed in this book has been pretty straightforward and, dare we say it, tame. Now it's time to push your

> *So far you've been counting your steps. Now it's time to make your steps count.*

thinking to the extremes. What's the wildest thing that you could do with the new you? What's the wildest direction you could go with your newly increasing physical fitness? Where would you go? What part of the world would you explore? Have fun with it. Whatever interests that you want to include in your life, no matter how extraordinary, there are others who feel the same way, people with similar passions and ideas—search them out on WalkStyles.com or another social forum.

You could also create new involvements (appropriate involvements, of course) with coworkers—maybe organize group hikes for your days off. You can go literally anywhere on the planet your two feet can take you. So why stay home? Life isn't a treadmill—it's an adventure.

It's best to choose goals that feel reachable—they should be a stretch, and you may not be quite sure right now how you're going to accomplish them, but at least you don't look at them and sink into despair, saying, "I could never do that!" A month or two ago, you probably never thought you could walk 10,000 steps a day!

> *Life isn't a treadmill—it's an adventure.*

In reality, we all want a lot of things—sometimes we just don't let ourselves dare to dream. This is the time to take that walk on the wild side and ask yourself what you would love. Often, the only thing standing in the way of our dreams is our own belief system. Lou Holtz, the famous football coach, once made a list of a hundred things he wanted to do before he died. One of them was "coach a national championship football team." He wrote the list at a time when his career was at its lowest point, and it seemed all but impossible to anyone but him that he would have the opportunity to ever do something like that. Of course, Lou Holtz went on to coach Notre Dame to a national championship. You can accomplish a lot more than you realize, if only you give yourself the power to do so.

Discipline

The question people often ask at this juncture is how to develop the discipline to follow through on the goals they set. Let's take a look at the word "discipline." Discipline simply means becoming a disciple to someone or something, a leader or perhaps a belief system. When you stop and think about it, we have a lot of discipline … to do things that aren't always in our best interest. When it comes to sitting down and snacking, many of us have all the discipline in the world! And when it comes to hitting the snooze button on the alarm clock two or three or four or five times after it goes off, we've got the discipline to do that too. You know what we're saying—we become disciplined to habits, good or bad.

The easiest way to accomplish great things with our lives is to discipline ourselves to great habits. And the easiest way to believe that we can discipline ourselves to great habits is to look back at our track record and see if we've done so. When you start seeing the success of achieving your daily dashboard count goals using the STAR™ process, you have learned you have the discipline to accomplish so much more. Again, it is taking steps towards your bigger goals. And you have now begun this process.

> *The easiest way to accomplish great things with our lives is to discipline ourselves to great habits.*

You have. You might have started off at 3,000 or 5,000 steps a day, and now you're at or near 10,000 steps a day. You might have had a few extra pounds around your waist, and now you see yourself slimming down, getting stronger and more attractive by the day. You might have seen that your work attitude wasn't the best—would *you* hire you? And now, because of your increased energy and vitality, you're a dream member of anybody's team. If you need proof that you can accomplish great things, take a look in the mirror. You already have.

To truly help yourself accomplish all your goals, keep in mind that journaling about your day and how you did accomplish your goals is extremely beneficial. It will give you a record to refer back to and a fun way to build daily memories. Your journal notes can be a great companion to your dashboard.

> *If you need proof that you can accomplish great things, take a look in the mirror. You already have.*

As we noted at the beginning of the book, this is all about you! Now, set your goal of using the STAR™ process, and let's get moving. Say it out loud again, "I count!"

Online Diagnostic Tool Input:

How would you assess your health at this time?
Do you feel you can start Setting, Tracking, Achieving, and Rewarding daily wellness goals?

Online Tracking Tools and Dashboard Input:

Ideas from this chapter to consider for the STAR™ process:

_____

_____

☆   ☆   ☆

Please go to WalkStyles.com to input the above.

Chapter 10:
I Count on the STAR™ Process

Daily Step #10: Continue to Set, Track, Achieve and Reward my daily goals.
Process: Use my tracking tools and my dashboard each day.
Healthy lifestyle goal: To live a long, happy and healthy life.

This book is your guide, and we hope it has inspired you to use the STAR™ process to set daily, achievable goals that help you become and stay healthier and happier, both physically and mentally. Again, if you keep stepping forward, good things will happen. That is why your daily step goal is non-negotiable!

The Online Diagnostic Tool

The diagnostic topics are at the end of each chapter, but the tool is online so you can get your score and other suggestions to support your wellness goals. Remember, this is not to be used in place of a physician's review but as a tool for you to have an understanding of your wellness.

As a member of WalkStyles.com, you can use the diagnostic tool to review your results, get comparisons from your baseline data, receive feedback on your progress, and help incorporate more healthy goals into your daily dashboard.

Online Tracking Tools

Your online tracking tools are available to you as part of your membership at WalkStyles.com. Here is where you set your step, nutrition, and other wellness goals. You can update and change your goals as appropriate. In addition, you can decide what goals (besides your step goal, of course) should be elevated to your dashboard.

The other feature of the tracking tools allows you to input your actual results. You will do this by either uploading your DashTrak® or manually entering your step information from your pedometer. You can enter your food and drink and get all your nutrition information in addition to your other wellness results. Thus, the online tracking tools is where you will utilize the Set and Track portion of the STAR™ process.

Finally, remember the importance of journaling in making your wellness goals a reality. You will find places to put your notes and thoughts when you are entering your actual results. This way you can capture what you are doing, how you were feeling or anything else important for you on your wellness journey.

Your Online Dashboard

As a member of WalkStyles.com, you will have your own personal dashboard. Here is where you will visually see your progress in achieving your step and other wellness goals. From the tracking tool input, your online dashboard will summarize your results and you will get stars based on your progress. Thus, your online dashboard is where you will utilize the Achieve and Reward portion of the STAR™ process. In addition, there are detailed levels of charts and graphs that are all about you!

My Dashboard Date *Sept. 30*

Nutrition
Meet my caloric goals
Goal *1800*
Actual *1683*
Reward ★

Health
Get sun everyday
Goal *15 minutes*
Actual *15 minutes*
Reward ★

Exercise
Do squats each day
Goal *5 squats*
Actual *8 squats*
Reward ★

STEPS: Goal *10,000* Actual *10,269* Reward ★
Distance: Goal *5 mi.* Actual *5 mi* Reward ★
Calories Burned: Goal *185* Actual *190* Reward ★

Others
Walk with friends
Goal *20 minutes*
Actual *one hour*
Reward ★

Blessings
Send a postcard
Goal *one*
Actual *none*
Reward

Workplace
Walk at lunch
Goal *20 minutes*
Actual *20 minutes*
Reward ★

For your complete dashboard and tracking system, go to WalkStyles.com.

If you are not a member of WalkStyles.com and you would like to create your own dashboard on paper, we have provided an example. Besides steps, you can decide what you want to track on your dashboard. We would recomend no more than seven goals. Of course, it is more powerful to have the interactive capabilities to help guide you through this process as you can keep records online and celebrate your success. However, we want you to be healthy whether you are a member or not!

> *When you get in the habit of achieving daily goals, you will feel the power of accomplishment!*

The Process

You now have the STAR™ process: Setting, Tracking, Achieving, and Rewarding. You can use this process for any goal in your life. Again, the one non-negotiable goal, from our perspective, is counting your steps. Our goal is to get you taking 10,000 steps or more a day. When you get in the habit of achieving daily goals, you will feel empowered. You can also use the STAR™ process to start setting bigger goals. Where would you like to go? How far can you go? These could be set around that promotion; that house;

that relationship. Remember, how you reach these bigger goals is by setting smaller goals that are going to lead you in the right direction.

Remember, do your daily goals for three weeks and they will become a habit. Do them for ten weeks and they will become part of your lifestyle.

We can't say it enough! Set, Track, Achieve, and Reward. And keep moving forward!

See, you count. You truly do! Shout it out loud. *I Count!*

We hope you have found a new discipline and a new commitment to your wellness. We also hope you learned that even if you miss a day, you can get back to stepping in the right direction. Focus on continuous improvement, don't overdo it, and never, ever take your eye off your dashboard. You can use this tool for the rest of your life. It is, after all, about you! Once again, out loud, "I count!"

We hope you have energized people around you to join you on your journey of wellness. We want to help you reach your desired destinations; we're just a click away at WalkStyles.com. You, your friends, family, and workplace are counting on you! Keep us up to date on your progress. We're counting on you, too!

Appendices:
Charts and Useful Information

Appendix A: Steps Conversion Chart

Table of Alternate Exercises and Their Step Equivalents Per Minute			
Calisthenics (light or moderate)	90	Kayaking (moderate)	125
Calisthenics (heavy effort)	200	Roller Skating (moderate)	175
Canoeing (2.5mph)	75	Rowing (leisurely)	90
Cross-Country Skiing (leisurely)	175	Rowing Machine (moderate)	175
Cross-Country Skiing (moderate)	200	Scuba Diving	190
Cross-Country Skiing (briskly)	225	Snow Skiing	175
Cycling (5mph)	100	Swimming (25 yds/ minute)	150
Cycling (10mph)	150	Swimming (50 yds/ minute)	175
Cycling (15mph, 5-minute mile)	250	Swimming (75 yds/ minute)	250
Elliptical (moderate)	225	Water Skiing	150
Elliptical (fast)	270	Weight Training (light to moderate)	75
Gardening (light)	100	Weight Training (vigorous)	150
Gardening (heavy)	150		

A more extensive step equivalent list is available at WalkStyles.com.

Appendix B: Calories Burned per Mile by Walking

Distance x weight = energy used (faster speed, more calories used per mile)

A slow-paced mile would take about 20 minutes, and you would complete three miles in a 60-minute period of time and about 6,000 steps. A faster pace of 15–17 minutes per mile will burn off more calories, and walking four 15-minute miles in an hour would equate to 364 calories for a 160-pound person and about 8,000 steps. (Use your pedometer for tracking distance and calories.)

Speed/ Pounds	100 lb	120 lb	140 lb	160 lb	180 lb	200 lb	220 lb	250 lb	275 lb	300 lb
2.0 mph	57	68	80	91	102	114	135	142	156	170
2.5 mph	55	65	76	87	98	109	120	136	150	164
3.0 mph	53	64	74	85	95	106	117	133	150	164
3.5 mph	52	62	73	83	94	104	114	130	143	156
4.0 mph	57	68	80	91	102	114	125	142	156	170
4.5 mph	64	76	89	102	115	127	140	159	175	191
5.0 mph	73	87	102	116	131	145	160	182	200	218

Source: Ainsworth BE, Haskell WL, Whitt MC, Irwin ML, Swartz AM, Strath SJ, O'Brien WL, Bassett DR Jr, Schmitz KH, Emplaincourt PO, Jacobs DR Jr, Leon AS. Compendium of Physical Activities: An update of activity codes and MET intensities. Medicine & Science in Sports & Exercise 2000;32 (Suppl):S498-S516.

Appendix C: Reward Suggestions for Achieving Goals

- Spend twenty minutes of time alone.
- Indulge in a bubble bath, steam or sauna
- Pamper yourself with a facial, massage, pedicure and/or manicure.
- Watch your favorite vintage movie with a friend.
- Shop for a new piece of clothing or shoes. (You'll need it when you lose weight!)
- Take your favorite book to the park and read.
- Pay yourself for steps, and save up for a fantastic weekend away.
- Attend a baseball, basketball, or football game with someone who loves the sport as much as you.
- Challenge a friend or family member, and enjoy the winnings.
- Participate in a charity walk.
- Buy yourself flowers, and put them on your desk or beside your bed.
- Spend time on your favorite hobby.
- Spend time in your garden.
- Buy that tool you have been putting off.
- Get your car detailed.
- Invite your friends over for a "poker night"
- Splurge on a golf or tennis lesson.
- Be creative!

You can tell us your favorite ways to reward yourself at WalkStyles.com.

Appendix D: Ways to Get Additional Steps

- Walking during commercial breaks of favorite TV shows
- Watching games, TV shows, or movies while on the treadmill
- Visiting art fairs and museums
- Shopping for:
  o groceries
  o gifts
  o clothing
- Hiking
- Visiting friends and family within walking distance
- Walking our favorite park during lunch hour
- Listening to a book on tape or music while:
  o Putting away laundry
  o Walking the dog
  o Emptying or filling the dishwasher
- Mowing the lawn (yes, it can be fun, lots of sunshine and great for steps!)
- Vacuuming our homes (not necessarily a favorite but it works!)
- Walking the golf course instead of using a cart
- Visiting a new city
- Parking far away from the store, office, train, etc.
- Having a walking meditation session
- Visiting the zoo
- Walking a beach …any beach…
- Dancing
- Using the stairs
- Walking versus using the moving sidewalks
- Volunteering and raising money for charity walks
- Jogging in place wherever we could be sitting (within reason)
- Walking to our favorite local restaurant or coffee shop
- Holding walking meetings
- Strolling hand in hand with someone we love

You can tell us how you get your steps in at WalkStyles.com.

Appendix E: Body Mass Index Chart

Know your BMI (body mass index). Your BMI is the relationship between how much you weigh and how tall you are. It's useful in determining if a person is at normal weight, overweight, or obese. After you have determined your BMI at WalkStyles.com, use this chart to see where you fit.

Risk of Associated Disease According to BMI and Waist Size

BMI		Waist less than or equal to 40 in. (men) or 35 in. (women)	Waist greater than 40 in. (men) or 35 in. (women)
18.5 or less	Underweight	--	N/A
18.5 - 24.9	Normal	--	N/A
25.0 – 29.9	Overweight	Increased	High
30.0 – 34.9	Obese	High	Very High
35.0 – 39.9	Obese	Very High	Very High
40 or greater	Extremely Obese	Extremely High	Extremely High

Source: "Body Mass Index Chart," Partnership for Healthy Weight Management, located at www.consumer.gov/weightloss/bmi.htm.

Appendix F: Sample Food and Calorie Logging Guide

Calorie Count	Food Item	Amount	Calories
Grains and Starches	Bagel, plain	1 med.	289
	Bread, whole wheat	1 slice	69
	Cereal, Cheerios	1 cup	111
	Cereal, Froot Loops	1 cup	118
	Couscous, cooked	1 cup	176
	Hamburger/Hot dog buns	1 bun	120
	Oatmeal, instant maple & brown sugar	1 packet	157
	Oatmeal, instant, plain	1 packet	97
	Pasta, cooked	1 cup	197
	Pita bread, white	1 x 6 ½"	165
	Potato, baked with skin	1 med	168
	Rice, white cooked	1 cup	205
	Tortilla, corn	1 x 6"	53
	Tortilla, flour	1 x 10"	228
Vegetables	Asparagus, cooked	½ cup	20
	Broccoli, cooked	½ cup	22
	Broccoli, raw	½ cup	30
	Carrots, cooked	½ cup	27
	Carrots, raw	1 cup	50
	Corn, frozen, cooked	½ cup	66
	Green beans, cooked	½ cup	22
	Mixed Veg., frozen, cooked	½ cup	59
	Peas, cooked	½ cup	62
	Spinach, raw	1 cup	7
	Spinach, cooked	½ cup	30

Fruits and Juices	Apple juice	1 cup	117
	Apple, raw with skin	1 med.	72
	Banana, raw	1 med.	105
	Cantaloupe, diced	1 cup	53
	Cranberry juice	1 cup	144
	Fruit cocktail, in juice	1 cup	109
	Grapes, red or green	1 cup	110
	Orange	1 med.	62
	Orange juice	1 cup	110
	Pinapple, canned in juice	1 cup	149
	Strawberries, whole	1 cup	46
	Watermelon, diced	1 cup	46
Beverages	Coffee, brewed	6 fl. Oz.	7
	Gatorade	8 fl. Oz	50
	Lemonade	8 fl. Oz.	131
	Tea, brewed	6 fl. Oz	2
	Soda, cola	12 fl. Oz.	155
	Beer	12 fl. Oz.	146
	Distilled alcohol (gin, rum, vodka, whiskey)	1.5 fl. Oz.	97
	Wine, white/red	4 fl. Oz.	80/85

A more extensive, interactive food guide is available at WalkStyles.com. A pound of fat equals 3,500 calories.

Meal	List Food	Size/Amount	Total Calories
Breakfast			
Breakfast			
Snack			
Lunch			
Lunch			
Lunch			
Snack			
Dinner			
Dinner			
Dinner			
Snack			
		Total Calories =	

Appendix G: Chart of Sleep Needed

Sleep Needs

"It is estimated that 50 to 70 million Americans chronically suffer from a disorder of sleep and wakefulness, hindering daily functioning and adversely affecting their health and longevity" (U.S. National Institute of Medicine). So, how much sleep do we really need to keep ourselves healthy? The following chart provides recommended hours of sleep per day. These are guidelines as sleep needs vary from person to person.

Group	Amount of Sleep Needed
Infants	About 16 hours per day of sleep
Babies and Toddlers	From 6 months to 3 years: between 10 to 14 hours per day
Children	Ages 3 to 6: between 10 to 12 hours of sleep Ages 6 to 9: about 10 hours of sleep Ages 9 to 12: about 9 hours of sleep
Teenagers	About 9 hours of sleep per night. Teens have trouble getting enough sleep not only because of their busy schedules, but also because they are biologically programmed to want to stay up later and sleep later in the morning, which usually doesn't mesh with school schedules.
Adults	For most adults, 7 to 8 hours a night appears to be the best amount of sleep, although some people may need as few as 5 hours or as many as 10 hours of sleep each night.
Older Adults	Current thought is that older adults need as much, if not more, sleep than middle-aged adults. Taking a midday nap may help.
Pregnant Women	During pregnancy, women may need a few more hours of sleep per night.

Source: HelpGuide.org, "Typical Sleep Needs Chart," available at http://www.helpguide.org/life/sleeping.htm.

References:

Chapter One

1. Statistics on obesity percentages – National Center for Health Statistics, Chartbook on Trends in the Health of Americans Health, United States 2006. Hyattsville, MD: Public Health Service, 2006.
2. *40% of Americans participate in no leisure time activity* – MMWR (Morbidity and Mortality Weekly Report). Vol. 54/No. 47. December 2, 2005.
3. *37% less chance of heart attack* – The New England Journal of Medicine. Vol. 338. January 8, 1998. pg 94-99.
4. *2,000 steps = 10 lb. weight loss per year* – "Cutting Calories and CO2." The Orange County Register. November 12, 2007.
5. "Belly Fat linked to an Increased Risk of Dementia." USA Today. March 27, 2008.
6. *14 year quote* – University of Cambridge and The Medical Research. Www.BBCNews.com. January 8, 2008.
7. *10,000 steps/Japan over 40 years ago* – "Feet for Life." The Society of Chiropodists and Podiatrists (Internet). June 2004.
8. *University of Tennessee study* – Fusell, James A. "Walk 10,000 Steps a Day and Count on Losing Weight," *SeaCoast online*. April 5, 2007.
9. *Amish Study* – "Physical Activity in an Old Order Amish Community." Medicine & Science Sports & Exercise (Internet). January 2004.
10. *Stanford University study on tracking steps* – "Pedometer Pushes People to Walk More." The Washington Post. November 20, 2007.

Chapter 2

11. *Dog obesity reference* – Orange County Register. February 17, 2007.
12. *One in three children diabetes* – "The Surgeon General's Call to Action to Prevent and Decrease Overweight and Obesity." United States Department of Health and Human Services. November 27, 2007.
13. National Sleep Foundation. "Employees Lacking in Sleep." The New York Times. March 3, 2008.

14. *Childhood obesity reference* – "F as in Fat: How Obesity Policies are Failing in America." <u>Trust for America's Health</u>. pg 3.
15. "The Surgeon General's Call to Action to Prevent and Decrease Overweight and Obesity." <u>United States Department of Health and Human Services</u>. November 27, 2007.

Chapter 5

16. Brosner, Robert J. and Deboral L. Caldron. "Health and High Performance." www.ExecutiveHealthCoach.com.

Chapter 6

17. "Friends help friends stay fat." <u>New England Journal of Medicine.</u> July 26, 2007.
18. *Kids walking to school* – <u>US News & World Report</u>. September 10, 2007. pg 6.

Chapter 7

19. *$285,000 for 1,000 employees* – "Financial Incentives Can Encourage Weight Loss." USA Today, September 10, 2007.
20. *Breakdown on health for every 100 workers* – "Characteristics of Successful Wellness Programs." <u>American Institute for Preventive Medicine (Internet)</u>. 2007.
21. *Research that confirmed incentives can help employees make lifestyle changes* – "Encouraging a Healthy Lifestyle in the Workplace." <u>Triangle Business Journal</u>. Feb. 1, 2008. pg 112.
22. The Washington Post *article on U.S. emissions and walking* – "Cutting Calories and CO2." <u>The Orange County Register</u>. November 12, 2007 .

Printed in the United States
144218LV00004B/2/P

9 780595 526192